Hip arthritis / hip pain explained.

Osteoarthritis in hips and rheumatoid arthritis in hips.

Including hip flexor pain, hip arthritis replacement surgery, exercises, treatments, physiotherapy and aids.

by

Robert Rymore

Published by IMB publishing 2014.

D1637082

1

Disclaimer

This book was written by the author as a guide to self-help. However, the author and/or publisher take no responsibility as to the correctness, timeliness and standard of the writings.

Any websites, service providers, books and devices suggested herein are only written as suggestions; the author and/or publisher do not endorse these items. Any repercussions resulting from their use are the reader's liability.

Furthermore, any links found in this book have been double-checked for functionality; however, any consequences resulting from using these links are the reader's own responsibility.

Any medications, exercises and/or medical gadgets mentioned in this book require your doctor's consultation, advice and prescription. Failure to abide by these terms is the reader's liability.

Lastly, the contents of this book are the author's own copyrighted material; use of any writings in this book without the author's consent is prohibited.

Table of Contents

Table of Contents

Table of Contents

Preface

Robert Rymore has been writing medical educational guides for 5 years now, and this guide on hip arthritis is one of his many. His books are well-researched, and written in easy-to-understand English that is void of any medical jargon. However, it is difficult for one to write on any medical subject without mentioning some medical terms. When these terms do get used in this book, they are well-explained in such a way that any reader will be at ease and in their comfort zone as they read through.

Hip arthritis is one of the leading debilitating medical conditions in the world, where the elderly, adults and even the young are affected. This book is aimed at thoroughly educating the reader on hip arthritis. It covers general anatomy of the hip, probable differential diagnosis of hip arthritis, the main pathology of hip arthritis, and how it can be managed from home. It also describes the different kinds of treatment available on the market to eliminate pain and to enhance the general functions of a sufferer.

A must-read for anyone who would like to understand more on what hip arthritis is.

Foreword

My colleague Robert never ceases to amaze me. His will and effort in writing medical educational guides is admirable. After having read the manuscript of this book, all I can say is "Spot on."

4 months ago, it was found that I had a labrum tear on my left hip. Nothing else was revealed on radiographical imaging, ultrasound and chiro adjustments among other avenues. Even though most tests did not show any immediate pathology, my pain got progressively worse, reducing my activity to zero running or cycling. My doctor advised me on arthroscopy, which I opted for. The results turned out to be a moderate osteoarthritis on the lateral side of my left hip joint.

Robert's book is relatable to my situation, as it explains thoroughly what I am dealing with. The anatomical orientation was excellent, since I never quite understood what the labrum was, and what moderate osteoarthritis meant. This book is amazing, I recommend it to anyone seeking knowledge on hip arthritis.

Robert, thank you for this read. It came through right on time.

Denise Marlon,
Nottingham 2014

Acknowledgements

With heartfelt gratitude, I would like to thank the following people for their assistance in making publishing of this book possible:

Pamela Kirstin,
Theresa R. Higgins,
Jason Moyra,
Adam G. Coventry,
Philip T. Maison,
Johanah S. Crawford,

And

My family, for their never-ending support

Introduction

The hip is one of the largest joints in the human body. It is also one of the largest axial weight bearers of the body, that allows locomotion from one point to another, and activities like running, sitting, squatting, and jumping. The hip is a ball-and-socket joint. Like a lock and key, the head of the thigh bone locks into a groove on the pelvic bone, the acetabulum, to form the hip joint. This construct is held in place by the supporting components of the hip joint, which consist of the labrum, ligaments and muscles. Like any other joint in the body, the hip has a neurovascular bundle, which supplies it with nutrients and sensation. However, the blood supply of the hip joint is peculiar, such that when it is injured, its recovery is severely compromised. This compromise, I must add, depends on the age of the patient.

Hip arthritis is the term used when the articulating surfaces of the hip joint rub against each other, corroding the articular cartilage. It is a painful condition in which the sufferer loses function and therefore productivity. According to the Centers for Disease Control and Prevention (CDC) in the United States, 50% of above-65 year olds have reported being diagnosed with arthritis. Also in the United States, 50 million adults have been reported to have some form of arthritis, i.e. rheumatoid arthritis, gout, reactive arthritis, osteoarthritis and septic arthritis to mention but a few. Projections for 2030 estimate that about 67 million Americans of 18 years of age and older are to be diagnosed with some form of arthritis.

Not only is the arthritis prevalence great in the United States, but its prevalence is on the rise everywhere else in the world.

According to Arthritis Research UK, more than 650,000 people in the U.K. have painful osteoarthritis of one or both hips. More than 10 million British adults are estimated to consult their GP yearly on arthritis-related complaints.

The disease is more prevalent in women than in men, of ages over 65, and of white ethnicity. Obesity also plays a major role in its development. Class III obese individuals have the highest risk of developing hip arthritis, followed by Class II, then class I. Generally, being overweight predisposes one to the development of hip arthritis, and moreover, any form of arthritis.

Inactivity is another factor that has been shown to increase the probability of developing hip arthritis. Other factors that are worth mentioning are lifestyle choices like smoking.

The hip joint is the second most affected weight-bearing joint, after the knee, and osteoarthritis is the most frequent arthritis subtype. Hip arthritis development, besides the already mentioned predisposing factors, and heredity, can affect any individual at any time. After its initial development, diagnosing the condition early and initiation of proper medications early will greatly reduce its progression.

Hip arthritis is diagnosed by multiple medical tests, though X-ray imaging is the most leading investigation due to its availability and cost. Other tests that can be performed include blood tests like erythrocyte sedimentation rate (ESR), full blood picture (FBP), and some biochemical tests like uric acid level checks, calcium and phosphate levels. Magnetic resonance imagings (MRIs) are top on the list, as they diagnose even soft tissue injuries including blood vessel infarctions. However, this imaging technique is expensive for both the patient and the service provider. Computer tomography scanning (CT scans), ultrasonography, arthroscopy and biopsy are some of the medical tests that can be performed. Once diagnosed, many modalities of treatment can be initiated to reduce pain and to improve function. Non-steroidal anti-inflammatory drugs (NSAIDs), glucosamine and chondroitin sulphate, and corticosteroid injections are the most used pharmacological preparations. Physiotherapy, yoga, acupuncture and chiropractics are some of the treatment activities that can be performed by patients at home, and or with help from the respective specialist. When conservative means of hip arthritis treatment fail to reach the desired effect, surgery can be considered where partial and total hip replacements are leading.

This book will take you through all the things that one should know and understand about hip arthritis. So, brace yourself for an informative expedition.

Chapter 1: Hip anatomy

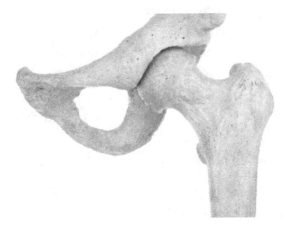

The picture above shows an anterior view of a human hip joint.

The human body is made up of the axial skeleton and the appendicular skeleton. The axial skeleton is the erect body parts that support the position of the body in space, like the spine. The appendicular skeleton comes from the term "appendage," which in this context means the upper and lower limbs and/or extremities. The hip joint, or coxa, is a ball-and-socket joint, comprising of two bones articulating together. The ball is formed by the femur (thigh bone) head, while the socket is formed from the acetabulum. The hip joint connects the axial skeleton to the appendicular skeleton.

The surfaces of the joint are covered by articular cartilage. Articular cartilage is a whitish, smooth and shiny substance, which covers the surface of any part of the body that is designated to be a joint.

One should not confuse the hip joint and the hip bone. The hip bone or os coxa, is formed by 2 sections of the pelvis that come

12

together during skeletal development. Each section of the pelvis, either on the right side or the left side, is made up of 3 bones that fuse together during puberty, namely the ilium, ischium and pubis. The 2 pelvic sections are joined anteriorly by the pubic symphysis, and posteriorly by the sacrum and coccyx, forming a single pelvis.

For one to completely understand the anatomy of the hip joint, it is necessary for us to go through each and every bone separately.

1) Femur

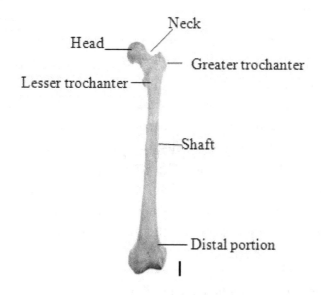

The femur is one of the long bones in the human body. It is located above the knee cap (patella) and the pelvis. The proximal part of the femur is formed by the head, which participates in formation of the hip joint, while the distal knobbed part participates in the knee joint formation. The length of the femur is called the shaft or diaphysis. The superior or proximal segment of the femur consists of the head, neck, greater and lesser

13

trochanters. The head and the neck of the femur are at a 30° angle, towards the medial (inward) direction. This angle in a newborn is large; however, it decreases with age. This angle is known as the CCD angle, standing for caput (head), cervical (neck) and diaphysis (shaft)-angle. The CCD angle can be decreased or increased abnormally in the presence of pathology, e.g. in fractures. When the CCD angle increases above the normal limit, it is known as coxa valgus; if it decreases, coxa vara. Treatment modalities in such cases aim at restoring the CCD angle, hence the weight-bearing position, without which pain and discomfort can persist.

The greater trochanter is a bony prominence that is located on the outward (lateral) side of the femur. It serves as an attachment site for the gluteus medius and minimus muscles. The lesser trochanter is located on the medial side of the proximal femur. It is the insertion site for the iliopsoas muscle. A line that appears like a ridge between the greater and lesser trochanters in front is called the inter-trochanteric line, while posteriorly, the intertrochanteric crest. The intertrochanteric line or crest is a point of weakness, since in the elderly, most fractures occur in this region. However, other sites of the femur can also be injured.

2) Pelvis

At birth, the pelvis is made up of 3 separate, primary bones: the ilium, the ischium and the pubis. These 3 bones are initially joined together by cartilage of the hyaline kind. These bones together form a hemi-section of the pelvis, what we call the hip bone. They are joined in a Y-shaped joint at the acetabulum, what is called a triradiate joint. When one views the pelvis of an adult, traces of the lines that once were joining the separate bones are not visible. Fusion of these bones occurs at ages 16-17 years, but complete ossification is done by 23-25 years of age.

1) Ilium

The ilium is the largest of the 3 bones that make a hip bone. It is a saucer-like bone: flat, with a shallow depression inside it. It has some large crests: 2 anterior (in front) and 2 posterior (at the back). The 2 anterior are the anterior superior iliac spine and the anterior inferior iliac spine, while the posterior 2 are the posterior superior iliac spine and the posterior inferior iliac spine. All the iliac spines are important anatomical landmarks. The top surface of the iliac bone is called the iliac crest. It consists of spongious bone, which is often harvested for bone grafting.

2) Ischium

The ischium is the part located at the back and inferior of the pelvis. It plays a role in supporting the sitting position, specifically the ischial tuberosity located on either side of the inner pelvis. The ischium, at the front of the pelvis, meets with the pubic bone to form rami, the ischiopubic rami. At the centre of the ischiopubic rami is the obturator foramen, which is the passageway of blood vessels and nerves from the pelvis to the lower limbs.

3) Pubis

The pubic bone is about 4-6 inches below the belly button. It is found in the front side of the pelvis. In women, the spongy urethra and uterus are located behind it. The pubic bone is divided into a body, the superior ramus and the inferior ramus. The body participates in formation of the acetabulum. The right and left hip bones are joined at the pubic symphysis, which is a cartilaginous joint that allows limited movement (an amphiarthrosis). The pubic symphysis is supported in place by 3 ligaments: the superior pubic, the arcuate pubic, and the interpubic disk.

4) Acetabulum

The acetabulum is a cup-like depression that forms the socket of a hip joint. It is formed by all 3 bones that form the hip bone. The acetabulum is covered by smooth cartilage, and at the centre has a pit, the fovea, where a ligament attaches the head of the femur to the acetabulum.

3) The hip joint

Besides being a ball-and-socket joint, the hip joint is a synovial joint. This means that it is surrounded by a joint capsule, which has a membrane, the synovial membrane, that produces synovial fluid. Synovial fluid can be thought of as brake fluid in a car, in the sense that it allows smooth, friction-free function of the hip joint. Synovial fluid function is further enhanced by the smooth articulating cartilage, which makes the hip joint movement effortless. The hip joint is one of the most stable joints in the human body. This stability is attributed to the following:

1) Ligaments

A ligament is a fibrous tissue band that connects a bone to a bone. In the hip joint, the iliofemoral, pubofemoral, ischiofemoral ligaments and the ligamentum teres all help in stabilizing the joint. These ligaments hold the femur head in the socket and prevent its dislodgment. Partial dislodgment of the femur head from the socket is known as subluxation, while a complete dislodgment is called a dislocation. Hip dislocations and subluxations are painful conditions that are orthopedic emergencies as they require immediate reduction to prevent injury of the hip blood vessels and nerves.

The hip ligaments support the hip anteriorly and hence the joint is more stable in extension and to some extent in flexion. However, when a force is applied at the knee with the hip at 90°, a posterior hip dislocation can result, the so-called dashboard injury.

2) Joint capsule
The joint capsule encircles the hip joint, from the intertrochanteric crest posteriorly, and the intertrochanteric line anteriorly. The joint capsule is a thick, white, and fibrous band that reinforces hip joint stability.

3) Muscles
Muscles around the hip joint also aid in hip joint stability. These muscles may completely cross over the hip joint and/or may have their origins or insertions around the hip joint. Whichever the case, hip joint muscles provide cushion, and thus protection to the hip joint. The hip muscles provide different kinds of movement at the hip, and the following muscle groups exist:

a) Hip extensors

Extending the hip also means straightening the hip. The muscles responsible for this movement are the gluteus maximus, and the hamstring muscles. Hamstrings are muscles found in the back of the thigh, namely the biceps femoris, the semitendinosus and the semimembranosus muscles.

b) Hip abductors

Abduction at the hip is movement in which you move your hip joints apart, such as when one stands with their feet wide apart. Hip abductor muscles include the gluteus minimus, the gluteus medius, and the extensor fasciae latae muscles.

c) Hip adductors

Adduction at the hip is the act of bringing the hip joints together, as in standing with your feet together. The muscles responsible for this action are the pectineus, the gracilis, and the adductor longus, brevis, and magnus muscles.

d) Hip rotators

These muscles allow the free inward or outward movement of the hip joint. Hip rotator muscles are further divided into internal and external hip rotators. Internal rotation of the hip is performed by some portion of the gluteus medius and the tensor fascia latae muscles. External rotators are the obturator internus and externus muscles, the inferior and superior gemellus muscles, and the quadriceps and piriformis muscles.

4) Labrum

The acetabular labrum is a fibrocartilage ring that encircles the acetabulum. The labrum acts as a shock absorber during weight bearing. The labrum increases stability to the hip joint by deepening the socket in which the femur head lodges. Some athletes who play sports like football, ballet and ice hockey to mention but a few may suffer from a labral tear. An individual with a labral tear usually complains of a locking feeling in the hip joint, which is associated with pain.

5) Bursa

A bursa is a fluid-filled sac that naturally occurs in areas of great pressure, e.g. where muscle tendons pass over bony protuberances. At the hip, bursae also help in supporting the stability of the joint. The greater trochanteric bursa is the largest at the hip. Since the greater trochanter is an attachment point for many muscles, the greater trochanteric bursa prevents muscle damage, as they glide over prominent bone of the greater trochanter. In some instances, a bursa may become irritated and inflamed, what is known as bursitis. Bursitis is a very painful condition, which often requires steroid injections to alleviate pain.

Chapter 2: Hip pain

Hip pain is any pain that occurs in or around the hip joint, although not every pain felt on the hip is from a hip-related problem. Pain at the hip may be referred from another region and in most cases from the lower back. Pain in the hip may result from several factors, and these factors can be any from a list of things like the bone, ligaments, labrum, bursa, neurovascular bundle, skin and other soft tissues.

Hip pain varies by certain specific parameters, which are explained as follows:

1) Duration of pain

Hip pain can be categorized as acute or chronic pain. Acute pain is one felt immediately, like after a hip fracture. Acute hip pain is specific in that it points to an immediate injury in the hip joint, e.g. a labral tear. Acute pain is often accompanied by anxiety, depression and stress.

Chronic hip pain occurs over a long period of time and may be tolerable, though it is very annoying. Chronic pain occurs with hip arthritis. As a disease like hip osteoarthritis progresses, the pain may become more intense and/or become constant. Chronic pain is also somewhat resistant to medical treatment. One might expect the pain to go away with medication use; however, breakthrough pain may be experienced by some sufferers. Whether the hip pain is acute or chronic, it always affects the sufferer's psychological being.

2) Causes of hip pain

Hip pain may be caused by many things, and these things can be remembered by the pneumonic "VITMIN D."

"V- Vascular"

Hip pain may arise from vascular insufficiency, e.g. in sufferers of diabetes mellitus or in sickle cell sufferers. This pain usually results from the femur head becoming infracted by inadequate blood supply and dying, which is known as avascular necrosis (AVN).

"I- Infection"

Hip pain can result from an infection such as tuberculosis of the hip joint, and other septic hip arthritis. Individuals that are immunologically compromised often suffer septic joint infections due to a staphylococcal infection.

"T-Tumour"

Hip pain may also result from a bone tumor at the hip and/or metastasis to the hip bones from a cancer originating from another organ. Patients with prostate cancer and breast cancer may have metastatic bone disease with the hip joint being affected. Pain at the hip due to cancer is often caused by pathological fractures. A pathological fracture is a fracture that occurs in an already diseased bone after a low-energy injury like falling off of the bed.

"M- Metabolic"

Metabolic diseases may be a reason for hip pain. Metabolic conditions that involve a lack of enzymes or an excess of one

21

particular substance may result in hip pain. These diseases include diabetes mellitus, Paget's disease, gout, systemic lupus erythematosus, osteoporosis and osteonecrosis.

"I- Inflammation"

The immune system is a system in the body that helps us fight off disease. It involves inflammatory cells, e.g. white blood cells, and inflammatory substances like tumor necrosis factor, leukotrienes and the complement system. In hypersensitive individuals, the immune system may attack its own tissues, and that can be one source of pain at the hip, e.g. in rheumatoid arthritis.

"N- Neuropathy"

Nerve injury by trauma, compression and/or degeneration due to age may also result in hip pain. Sciatica is one example that affects many people over 40 worldwide.

"D- Degeneration"

Hip joint degeneration is another source of pain. Since a degenerative condition requires many years for it to develop and progress, hip degenerative conditions often affect individuals over 30 years old. Diseases like post-traumatic hip arthritis, osteoarthritis, and degenerative joint disease are examples of sources of pain at the hip.

3) Pain intensity

The intensity of hip pain varies from an ache to a sharp, stabbing or throbbing pain. Pain intensity often correlates with the acuteness of the condition. Acute hip pain is usually sharp and throbbing, while chronic pain is often dull, achy and tolerable. However, even with chronic pain, an acute episode may occur, resulting in a stabbing pain in a background of dull aches.

Pain intensity can be classified as mild, moderate and severe. It is common to use a numeric score from 0-10 for pain intensity estimation. Pain that is less than or equal to 4 is considered mild. Pain between 5 and 6 is said to be moderate, while pain scaled at 7 and more is classified as severe. Most patients with severe hip pain require hospital admission and/or have a history of several hospital admissions due to pain.

4) Others

Hip pain classification also includes other criteria like the specific time at which the pain occurs e.g. night time. The things that alleviate or aggravate the symptoms are also criteria. Rest may temporarily relieve arthritic pain, while cooling with an ice pack can help an inflammatory kind of pain. Pain due to cancer often does not respond to simple pain medications and may require narcotic-based medications like morphine. The associative symptoms to the hip pain should be reported. These may often point to the main cause of hip pain, e.g. fever for a septic hip joint, or severe night sweating with a tuberculous hip.

Hip pain severity is to some extent age-specific, as the causes of hip pain are also age-specific. A septic hip joint may be frequent in neonates, and may point to immunosuppression if it develops in an adult. A hip fracture may be frequent in the elderly, but when it occurs in children may point to an underlying bone disease like rickets. Such age-specific hip pain epidemiology is very important, as a patient may be complaining of only hip pain, when the main disease is probably systemic.

Hip pain can be categorized into age groups. Individuals below 16 years of age are considered to be children, and those from 16-65 years are adults, while over 65-year-olds are classified as elderly.

a) Hip pain in the elderly

At an elderly age, most people have age-related ailments. These include osteoporosis and osteomalacia. Women over 65 years of age are a decade or two post-menopause, so the hormones progesterone and estrogen are lower than in their younger days. Estrogen and progesterone play a role in bone development, as they boost body cells that add calcium to bones for strength. In the absence of the hormones, these body cells lose the ability to lay down new bone, leading to activation of a different kind of cell that removes calcium from bones. Loss of calcium will result in a weaker bone that has a low density. Due to this reason, the elderly are often at risk of getting hip fractures. Hip fractures affect women more than men. According to the CDC, in 2010 about 258,000 hospital admissions occurred due to hip fractures in people over 65 years of age. Furthermore, the CDC projects that in 2030, hip fractures will have increased by 12% in this age group.

In over-65s, cancer is also a frequent diagnosis, such that complications of cancer also result in hip pain. Diseases like arthritis are also more evident in this age group. In the hip, osteoarthritis is the leading form of arthritis, followed by rheumatoid arthritis. Other forms of arthritis like reactive arthritis and gout may also occur. Other conditions like hypertension, diabetes mellitus, atherosclerosis and vascular insufficiency are also high in this age group. These conditions make management of hip pain in the elderly a challenge, as they tend to have a higher risk of complications, e.g. pressure sores and thrombosis. It is also important to note that in over-65s, their daily activity and exercise is low, rendering them more vulnerable to activity-related conditions like obesity. Obesity has a negative effect on any joint in the body, and for a large, weight-bearing joint like the hip, arthritis is bound to start sooner or later. However, analgesics, physiotherapy, conservative and surgical managements can be opted for, depending on the condition.

2) Adults' hip pain

Hip pain in adults points to conditions related to activity or overuse. These conditions include hip arthritis, hip fractures, bursitis, tendonitis, muscle strain, osteonecrosis and tumors. Furthermore, referred pain from the lower back is common in adults. Other reasons for hip pain involve groin hernia in men, while in women referred pain from a pelvic inflammatory disease is common. This age group is also a sexually active group and chronic pain of the reproductive organs can be referred to the hips, e.g. sexually transmitted diseases. Whatever the diagnosis, having a correct examination by a doctor and having medical tests performed on time will help to treat more immediate conditions early.

3) Hip pain during pregnancy

Hip pain during pregnancy is common. It is usually attributed to the pelvic girdle instability, where the symphysis pubic dysfunction (SPD), diastasis of the symphysis, and pelvic girdle pain deserve a mention.

As pregnancy progresses, hip pain and back pain become more apparent. As the baby grows, the uterus grows up to about one thousand times its original size. The American College of Obstetricians and Gynecologists states that if such an increase in size and weight is centered in a single location, the balance of the body in space changes, thus causing discomfort. As the belly grows, a pregnant woman appears more and more tipped over backwards. This tipping over causes a strain on muscle groups that otherwise are not normally stretched, resulting in pain.

The pregnancy hormones progesterone and relaxin increase laxity of joint ligaments. This is necessary during pregnancy so as to allow enough room for the fetus, and to increase the pelvic size in preparation for child birth. Ligaments are fibrous bands that function to stabilize joints. During pregnancy, the lax ligaments render most joints unstable, the hip included. This is why hip pain and lower back pain are common in pregnant women. Hip pain during pregnancy shows up earlier and earlier with each subsequent pregnancy.

Hip pain during pregnancy may also be due to sleeping on one side, which is true in the third trimester. Individuals who had a prior hip pain may also experience increased pain intensity. The same applies to women who were obese before becoming pregnant. With any pregnancy, women tend to gain more weight, and adding weight to an already overweight body will quicken the symptom presentation for hip pain due to arthritis.

Exercises and yoga during pregnancy help in relieving hip pain (see the chapter on treatment for hip pain).

4) Pain in children

Hip pain in children is often associated with infections, congenital conditions and mechanical instability of the hip joint. Some congenital hip dysplasias predispose children to pain even before they reach the walking age. A septic hip joint is common in children and is an orthopedic emergency. Children with a septic hip are irritable, avoid using the affected hip, and almost always run a fever in the acute phase. At the doctor's, an emergency opening of the hip joint is required so as to evacuate pus and wash the joint up, which is called an arthrotomy. If an arthrotomy is not performed, in as little as two days the joint cartilage can be completely eroded, resulting in a severe arthritis in a child. As the child grows, such an early, severe arthritis has a bad prognosis.

Other probable infections of the hip in a child include a psoas muscle abscess and osteomyelitis of the femur head or pelvis. Mechanical conditions like a slipped capital femoral epiphysis (SCFE), Leg-Calve-Perthes disease, and sickle-cell disease may cause AVN of the femur head at the hip, and therefore pain. These cause hip pain during walking and a child may also initially report the pain in the knee (take note as this is just referred pain).

Septic arthritis is frequent in 0-6-year-olds, while Perthes disease peaks at 5-7 years, but generally is typical in ages 3-12 years. SCFE usually occurs in adolescent children of 12-16 years, with a male to female ratio of 1.5:1.

Child obesity is also a growing diagnosis. It increases the risk of children developing any one of the mentioned conditions.

5) In cats and dogs

Cats and dogs are part of our daily lives, and many households have a cat or a dog, or both. It only seemed fair to include knowledge on our pets in this book as far as hip pain is concerned.

Dogs of any age may suffer from hip arthritis. Unlike in humans, hip arthritis in dogs is not confined to adults and the elderly. Dogs with an inherited disease like hip dysplasia or osteochondrosis often suffer from hip arthritis. Infections and autoimmune diseases also play a role in hip pain in dogs. Dogs may develop hip pain after an injury. Signs like limping, altered gait, rapid panting, refusal to lie down or sleep, and running away when touched in certain areas are markers that your dog may be having hip pain. One out of five dogs may suffer from osteoarthritis in their lifetime. Large dogs and breeds are affected more, compared to small breeds like Chihuahuas. Obesity of any breed also predisposes to hip pain development. A dog with hip pain usually changes behavior. It becomes less active, has a limp and is evidently wincing with pain. Other conditions like cancer and back pain are also contributory to hip pain in dogs. An X-ray is necessary, and usually bony spurs or osteophytes are common findings in osteoarthritic dogs. Walking your dog as a means of exercise, and weight loss to an obese dog are helpful in the treatment of hip pain in dogs. Swimming as an exercise is a good choice, as water will make the dog feel light in space, thus enhancing its ability to move the affected joints.

Cats, on the other hand, do suffer from arthritis in their elderly age. However, the clinical picture is not as evident as in humans or dogs. Cats tend to hide their pain; this may be some sort of a survival instinct. In a study carried out in 2002, 90% of over-12-year-old cats had signs of arthritis on X-rays. At present, the causes of cat arthritis are unknown, but I suppose the usual, prime suspects are the likes of hip dysplasia, trauma and obesity. A cat owner should watch out for reduced activity, reduced mobility and altered grooming. An X-ray will diagnose arthritis in a cat, and a cat owner can suggest an X-ray at the vet's if they suspect their cat to be arthritic.

Chapter 3: Differentials of hip pain

Hip pain, as we have read in the previous chapter, can be due to a lot of medical conditions. For any treatment to be effective, a correct diagnosis for the hip pain should be made. A correct diagnosis of the cause hip pain is best made by a qualified medical doctor - to be on the safe side, doctors who deal with the hip on a daily basis like orthopedic specialists, rheumatologists or sports medicine specialists are best. A general practitioner who deals with general medical conditions might miss specific differential diagnoses to hip pain.

Differential diagnoses of hip pain are all the probable conditions that are specific to certain signs and symptoms that any patient may present with. From the list of differential diagnoses, medical tests are done to best evaluate the patient's clinical picture, after which a correct diagnosis should be made. This chapter will discuss a number of differential diagnoses to hip pain, their signs and symptoms, and how they can be correctly diagnosed and treated.

1) Hip dysplasia

The exact cause of hip dysplasia is unknown. However, its development is said to be multifactorial. Hip dysplasia, developmental dysplasia of the hip (DDH), or congenital dysplasia of the hip (CDH) mean one and the same thing. DDH is a developmental abnormality of the hip joint, where the acetabulum 'cup' is shallow and does not hold the femur head securely in place. Genetics and the hormone relaxin play a role in congenital development of the disease. Acquired forms of the disease result from swaddling infants, and placing babies in strange positions in a pram or car seat. Risk factors to its development include gender, breech presentation at birth, and a family history of hip dysplasia.

The exact time at which the condition develops is not known. Soon after birth the hip joint is cartilaginous in nature. The hip bone is still in its 3 separate bones, with the acetabulum appearing in a triradiate form. The femur head is still an epiphysis, and the greater and lesser trochanters are visualized as apophyses. The deep cup shape of the acetabulum develops due to the position of the femur head on the hip bone. If for some reason the femur head is not in its rightful position, the acetabulum will be shallow, with a new acetabulum forming elsewhere on the hip bone. This is known as a congenital hip dislocation. Pathology in ligaments that hold the femur head in its rightful place may also result in hip dysplasia. Whenever the femur head is not well secured in its socket, it tends to get subluxed or dislocated. Hip dysplasia ranges from an undetectable form, which often shows itself at an adult age as early arthritis, to maybe a hip anomaly with a completely dislocated hip. This condition occurs eight times more in females than males, and can affect both hips.

Symptoms

A baby with hip dysplasia has a hip that feels loose and can easily be dislocated during examination. During routine baby screening for hip dysplasia, a doctor purposefully dislocates and reduces the hip of a baby, as a way to check its stability. This testing is performed by means of the Ortolani test and Barlow maneuver. In the U.K., the term "clicky hips" is used to define the 'click' and 'cluck' that is heard when the Ortolani test and Barlow maneuver are positive.

A child with hip dysplasia has a lower limb length discrepancy, only if one hip is affected; otherwise when the problem is bilateral, limb length will be the same. Other symptoms include extra skin on the inside of the affected thigh, which makes the inguinal skin folds appear to be asymmetrical. Once a baby starts waking, they often walk on tip-toes, and have a limping or waddling gait.

Hip dysplasia is diagnosed by a doctor after performing a thorough physical examination. Imaging tests like ultrasound and X-rays are often performed. Ultrasound gives better results during the period when the joint is still cartilaginous in nature. Once diagnosed, treatment should be initiated. Treatment for hip dysplasia involves reducing the femur head into the true acetabulum, and holding it in place while the child grows. Holding of a reduced hip position depends on the patient's age. For children below six months of age, a Pavlik harness is often used to hold the lower limbs in an abducted position. A hip spica is used in babies over 6 months to 6 years of age. A hip spica is a type of a cast that is applied on both lower limbs of the child and the pelvis, fashioned to look like a trouser made from a cast. However, care has to be taken to prevent the cast from getting wet, and also to prevent development of pressure sores. The aim of hip dysplasia treatment is to treat it as early as possible. If early treatment is given, conservative treatment is often adequate. However, when symptoms present late, surgery is often indicated. Surgery involves corrective osteotomies and total hip replacements. A child with a missed hip dysplasia diagnosis will always suffer from chronic hip pain as an adult. Early arthritis development is the frequent complication for this condition.

Always seek help from doctors if you think your child's hips are not normal.

2) Piriformis syndrome

The piriformis muscle, as we learned from the previous chapter, is an external rotator of the hip. Under this muscle is where the sciatic nerve passes through from the pelvis to the lower limbs. Piriformis syndrome is a neuromuscular condition which is caused by the piriformis muscle compressing on the sciatic nerve. The piriformis syndrome may occur due to overuse of the rotator muscles of the hip and/or variations of the muscle and nerve position. This condition is a form of a nerve entrapment. Individuals like runners and cyclists, who have forward-moving activities, are predisposed to developing the disease. This can be due to overuse and fatigue of the piriformis muscle, which leads to spasm and/or hypertrophy of this muscle with consequent reduction of space for the sciatic nerve to pass.

Piriformis syndrome should be differentiated from sciatica. Sciatica is a nerve root compression syndrome that occurs due to spinal stenosis or herniated disk problems. The piriformis stretch test can be performed to mimic how the muscle compresses on the sciatic nerve, while the straight leg raising test can be performed for nerve root compression at the spinal level.

Symptoms

Pain in the gluteal region and the hip is one complaint often heard from sufferers. Also, tingling sensations and numbness in lower limbs and along the path of the sciatic nerve are often reported.

Diagnosis of this condition initially relies on a complete physical examination by a physician, followed by imaging tests. However, no imaging can diagnose this condition accurately. X-rays, MRIs and nerve conduction tests are performed to exclude other diseases from the diagnosis.

Treatment for piriformis syndrome is best provided by an experienced sports medicine specialist or a physiotherapist. These two will have knowledge as to the kind of exercises that you would need to perform in order to stretch the muscle. Strengthening exercises for other hip muscles like the hip extensors, abductors and external rotators will be helpful. Pain relief medications like NSAIDs, corticosteroid injections and ultrasound or shockwave procedures can be given. However, due to the deep position of the muscle and nerve, injections are best given with CT or ultrasound guidance. If all else fails, a nerve exploration surgery can be performed. Not only the piriformis muscle can compress on the sciatic nerve; other muscles and free-existing fibrous bands can too.

3) Flexor hip pain

Flexor hip pain occurs due to overuse of the flexor muscle group of the hip. Hip flexors allow you to lift your knees, and to flex or bend your waist. Athletes, soccer players and kick boxers are prone to hip flexor injuries that result in hip pain. Flexor hip pain is a sharp pain that is felt at the groin, where the thigh meets the pelvis. The iliopsoas muscle is the most commonly injured muscle in flexor hip pain. Repetitive motion of lifting the knees, like in most soccer practices, can result in tearing of flexor muscles. The tear may be partial, with slight pain and minimal disability, or the injury can be complete with severe loss of function.

Flexor hip injury can be graded into three categories, by the extent to which the muscle fibers are torn.

Grade 1 - minimal muscle fibers are injured

Grade 2 - a significant amount of muscle fibers are torn

Grade 3 - all muscle fibers are torn

Most common injuries are of the grade 2 type.

Over stretching flexor muscles to a range that is not usually reached can predispose one to this condition. It is thus of utmost importance to warm up adequately before any activities.

Symptoms

Sudden groin pain with an accompanying pulling sensation in front of the hip is a typical presentation. In severe cases, individuals may have muscle cramps with muscle spasm and weakness. In complete muscle tears, there is associated inability to continue with activity. Swelling, tenderness, and hyperemia can be seen, usually in the morning after injury. In severe cases, a hematoma and obvious deformity are visible.

Diagnosis of flexor hip pain can be confirmed by a physical examination. Imaging like X-rays, CT scans, MRI and ultrasound can be done to substantiate the diagnosis and/or to exclude other medical conditions. Treatment includes massage, ice or heat therapy, joint immobilization by the use of crutches or a walker, NSAIDs, ultrasound therapy and physiotherapy.

4) Iliotibial band syndrome

The iliotibial band is a thick, fibrous tissue that runs from the hip to the knee, on the lateral side of the thigh. The iliotibial band provides stability to both the hip and the knee joints. In some situations, this band is tight and taut, such that it limits free movement during activity and rubs against the bone when the hip or the knee is flexed. Due to this rubbing, the iliotibial band syndrome is also known as the iliotibial band friction syndrome. This syndrome is a possible diagnosis for hip pain, since a tight band will rub against the greater trochanter at the hip, resulting in its inflammation and pain. However, most sufferers of this syndrome complain of pain on the lateral surface of the knee, where the band rubs against the lateral femoral condyle. Bowlegs, increased outward rotation of the foot, uneven leg length, and high or low arches of the foot are risk factors to developing iliotibial band syndrome. In the U.S., this syndrome is common in long distance runners, with an incidence of 4.3-7.5% in this group of individuals. Tennis players and military recruits are also among individuals who are prone to developing the iliotibial band syndrome. This condition affects adults, with an equal distribution among men and women.

Symptoms

Pain that is localized at the greater trochanter is specific. However, a majority of sufferers feel pain on the lateral side of the knee. The pain is associated with activity and intensifies at an incline.

During local examination, a tender point can be found at the greater trochanter or above the lateral femoral condyle. A modified Thomas test can be performed, which is usually positive with a correct diagnosis of this syndrome. Laboratory tests for rheumatoid arthritis should be performed. Imaging tests are not really required, but if other conditions are suspected, imaging can be done for differential purposes.

Physiotherapy stretches and exercises are required on the treatment plan, although other modalities include NSAIDs and local steroid injections. If after conservative treatment no effect is achieved, tendon elongation surgery can be performed. Other surgeries that can be done involve osteotomy of the lateral femoral condyle, and a posterior release of the iliotibial band.

5) Cancer hip pain

Cancer is a mass or lump of cells formed from cells that divide abnormally. Cancer can be divided into benign and metastatic. Benign cancers are confined to one area, are slow-progressing, and do not spread to other body regions. Cancer can be classified by the cells in which it originates from, e.g. bone tissue, muscles and skin, to mention but a few. At the hip, cancer is often of bone origin. The different bone cancers that can result in hip pain have age-specific epidemiology. In children, bone cysts are frequent at the hip. These bone cysts can be curetted and bone grafted. In other instances, a local steroid injection can be carried out directly into the cyst. Bone cyst prognosis is usually good, although at times patients visit the doctor when they've already suffered a pathological fracture.

In teenagers, osteosarcoma at the hip may be a source of hip pain. Osteosarcoma is a very aggressive metastatic cancer of the bones, which is fast progressing. Most cases of osteosarcoma end up with an amputation or a disarticulation, before radiation or chemotherapy is initiated. In the elderly, multiple myeloma and chondrosarcoma are frequent causes of hip pain. In most cancers, the cause is unknown, but heredity, mutations, and environmental factors are among the suspected.

Symptoms

Pain in the area of cancer is the most common complaint. This pain is achy, and often wakes a sufferer up at night. Severe hip pain may result when a pathological fracture occurs. Metastatic cancer will have systemic symptoms like fever, fatigue, night sweats, loss of appetite and insomnia.

Diagnosis includes epidemiological findings, demographics, physical examination, laboratory and imaging tests. Physical examination may yield a tender swelling, which is non-mobile and soft, at times hard. X-ray will reveal a lytic, blastic, or mixed type bone lesion, which gives a high suspicion of bone cancer. Other specific findings on X-ray are the Codman triangle, soap bubbles appearance and/or a moth-eaten one. A full body scan may be helpful to locate other areas that could have been affected by the cancer. A definitive diagnosis for any cancer can only be yielded by taking a biopsy, with consequent histopathology tests. Many kinds of biopsies exist. Fine-needle biopsy (FNB) can be done under MRI, CT or ultrasound guidance. Open biopsy can also be performed. If an open biopsy is done in a well-equipped centre, histopathology results can be received intra-operatively, which aids the surgeon in performing the next step, e.g. total cancer excision.

Benign hip cancers have a better prognosis than metastatic ones. However, some benign cancers run a risk of becoming metastatic over time. Cancer treatment generally involves chemotherapy, radiotherapy, bone marrow transplant, and combinations of limb salvage and amputations. Other supportive treatments are given symptomatically, e.g. blood transfusions for an anaemic cancer. Pain management is the most challenging, and palliative care.

6) Tattoo hip pain

Hip tattoo pain is pain experienced at the hip following a tattoo at the hip. A tattoo at the hip is one of the most painful tattoos to have done, mainly because the needles are close to the bone in that location.

Tattoos are often put as a way of expression. A tattoo often is meant to express one's personality, their interest in something, and/or their love for something. Tattoos that are done on the hips are frequent in women. Tattooing an area with little subcutaneous fat predisposes one to pain following being tattooed. This pain is usually accompanied by itching, though one should avoid scratching. Tattoo pain lasts for about a week; however, it depends on the design, size, color and shade.

Tattoo pain feels like being burned and poked at the same time. The shading hurts more than the outlines. On the pain scale, tattoos that are done on the hip, ribcage, genitals, nipple, lips and inner thighs are the most painful. However, pain measurement is dependent on an individual's threshold for pain toleration. For starters, a tattoo on the upper arm, bottom, forearm or calf is not as painful and often is chosen by first-timers.

Tips before having a tattoo at the hip

- Take someone with you, to chat to while you have your tattoo done.

- Use moisturizing lotion on the site where the tattoo is to be applied 2-3 weeks beforehand.

- Drink plenty of fluids before having a tattoo.

- Find out if you are allergic to any pigments or dyes beforehand.

- Consult your doctor before getting a tattoo if you are taking any blood thinning medications. Bleeding may be a complication in this case after having your tattoo.

- Keep clothes away from a tattoo soon after having it done and the week after; rubbing against the tattoo is not recommended.

- Have a licensed tattooist do the job for you; make sure the equipment used is adequately sterilized. Diseases like hepatitis B can be spread through needle pricks.

7) Fibromyalgia

Fibromyalgia is a condition characterized by widely distributed musculoskeletal pain. Its cause is unknown; however, it is complex in origin and results in chronic pain disorders. Fibromyalgia is also known as fibrositis, fibromyositis and fibromyalgia syndrome. It consists of multiple tender points, abnormal processing of pressure, fatigue, insomnia and psychological stress. Fibromyositis is debilitating; in severe cases it can lead to zero activity.

Tender points in fibrositis involve the neck, shoulders, back, hips, arms and legs. Therefore, hip pain may arise due to its occurrence. Fibrositis is associated with other diseases like systemic lupus erythematosus and rheumatoid arthritis. Risk factors to its developments include the female gender, rheumatic disease and a family history. The CDC showed that in 2005 about 5 million adults in the U.S. suffered from fibromyalgia and that its prevalence is 2%. Average hospital expenditures per individual that suffers from fibromyalgia ranges between $3,400 - $3,600, with an annual estimation of close to $6,000. People with fibrositis react strongly to pressure and pain, which any normal individual would find not painful.

Symptoms

Pain in fibromyalgia is generalized to all body parts and is chronic. All these body parts may present with pain of varying intensities. Pain in fibrositis is often defined as sharp, stabbing, shooting, twitching and at times throbbing. Associated neurological feelings like numbness and tingling sensations may be reported. Pain is worse during the mornings, where it's accompanied by stiffness. Physical inactivity, cold weather, and stress may worsen the condition. Many patients with fibromyalgia also report sleep disturbances, fatigue, headaches, lack of concentration, skin problems, depression, poor memory and ringing in their ears. These symptoms accumulate over time, but at times are triggered by physical trauma, surgery, stress, or an infection.

Diagnosis of fibromyositis is made by means of closely following a patient's history, symptoms and signs. A physical examination may also reveal the tender points. Laboratory tests and X-rays are often negative. However, most doctors are not experienced with fibromyalgia so a patient is often diagnosed after several years of wasted money in laboratory and imaging tests.

Fibrositis has no cure. Its treatment is based on symptomatic therapy and improving the patient's comfort. It relies on medications and self-care. Medications often used for its treatment are analgesics like Tylenol, Ultram, NSAIDs, antidepressants, and anti-seizure drugs. Psychological support will be required to reduce stress. Regular physiotherapy, eating healthy meals and getting enough sleep are some of the self-care treatment measures. Some alternative treatments like yoga, massage and acupuncture can also be considered.

Fibromyalgia is a challenging disease that needs more awareness, research and support. Since there is no cure for fibromyalgia, its prognosis is difficult to measure and is individual-based. However, every individual can try to make their prognosis better by following management plans.

8) Endometriosis

The tissue that lines the inside of the uterus is called the endometrium. Endometriosis is when this tissue type grows in areas outside of the uterus, e.g. the ovaries, oviducts and other structures of the pelvis. Endometriosis is associated with severe low abdominal pain and pelvic pain, associated with the monthly menstrual cycle. About 5-10% of women suffer from this condition.

In a healthy woman, hormones cause the endometrial lining of the uterus to hypertrophy in preparation for fertilization of the ova to take place. When fertilization does not occur, the endometrium is shed as a menstrual period every month. In endometriosis, the other locations where the endometrial tissues have grown also respond to hormonal changes. These tissues also shed and bleed as in a monthly period. Bleeding in endometriosis is not allowed to escape, resulting in inflammation of tissues, and at times cyst formation. The accumulated blood will cause tissues of the body to stick together by means of fibrous tissues called adhesions.

The cause of endometriosis is unknown; however, genetics and the seeding theory are the most talked of.

Symptoms

Symptoms of endometriosis include painful menstrual periods, pain during sexual activity, heavy periods, and pain with bowel movements during periods, abdominal pain, back pain, leg pain, emotional stress, fatigue and headaches. Endometriosis pain feels like a sudden on-and-off cramp. This pain is sharp, below the belly button and just above the groin. The pain is unpredictable; it is on and off as it wishes with no specific timing. Endometriosis pain often spreads down to the hip and leg, causing difficulties in walking. Adhesions that result in endometriosis may trap the sciatic nerve, such that tingling sensations and numbness along the sciatic nerve's route is common.

Endometriosis is a clinical diagnosis, and a laparoscopy can substantiate its presence. Laparoscopy is a type of a medical investigation where, under anesthesia, a doctor introduces a tube with a light and camera at the end into the abdomen through a very small incision. The thin tube is moved around in the abdomen as the doctor views the interior of the abdomen on a screen monitor.

Like fibromyalgia, endometriosis has no cure. Its treatment goals are to relieve the patient's symptoms thus it's a symptomatic treatment. Pain medications are prescribed. Hormone therapy with the use of birth control pills is another treatment option. Often, infertility is a complication of this medical condition. In severe cases, removal of the uterus and both ovaries may be required to stop the pain symptoms.

Sufferers of endometriosis may complain of pain all over the joints of the body (the so-called endometriosis joint pain). However, the hip is the most common and should be excluded from differentials of hip pain. Whether or not hip pain is a direct symptom of endometriosis is not certain.

9) Scoliosis

The term scoliosis is Greek for 'crooked.' Scoliosis is a back condition where the vertebral bones are curved and crooked in areas where they otherwise should be straight. In scoliosis, the back bends sideways. Scoliosis develops in older children of ages 9-15 years, during the growth spurt at puberty. Scoliosis is a progressive condition in children; its prognosis is worse if it starts at a very young age. It is not only confined to children; scoliosis can develop in adults as an acquired type.

Classification of scoliosis

a) Postural or functional scoliosis - not a true scoliosis. The back appears to be scoliotic, but once the affected individual straightens or changes position, it goes away. Postural scoliosis may occur due to other conditions like leg length discrepancies or muscle spasm.

b) Structural scoliosis - the back is permanently curved to the side, such that even if the person straightens or changes position, it remains the same. Structural scoliosis can further be divided into subgroups by the main cause:

❖ Neuromuscular diseases like muscular dystrophy result in weak muscles of the back, which cannot hold the body in an erect position. Other neurological conditions like cerebral palsy and polio may also result in this kind of scoliosis.

❖ Congenital scoliosis - the vertebral bones in this case are abnormal since birth, resulting in poor development as the child grows.

❖ Osteopathic scoliosis - results when the vertebral bones have abnormalities.

❖ Idiopathic scoliosis - when the cause of scoliosis is unknown, it is referred to as idiopathic. Idiopathic scoliosis is the most frequent type, present in 80% of all scoliosis cases.

Scoliosis development is not known, including how or why it develops, but researchers think physical abnormalities, coordination problems, and biological factors like defective proteins are responsible for its occurrence. 2-3% of the population has scoliosis; this is about 6 million people in the U.S. Girls are affected more than boys.

43

Scoliosis can be further graded by the affected age;

❖ Infantile - 3 years and below

❖ Juvenile - 4-9 years of age

❖ Adolescent - over 10 years of age

Symptoms

Signs of scoliosis include a tilted pelvis with uneven hips, uneven shoulders, and a 'C' or 'S' curve of the spine. Scoliosis is more visible when the Adam's forward bending test is performed. During this test, an individual bends to touch the toes, maintaining the legs in a straight position. Due to the imbalance in muscles of the back, most patients complain of pain which ranges from mild to severe. Back pain and hip pain may be reported. The back develops a bulge at the back of the chest and in severe cases the thoracic organs like the heart and lungs may be compressed, resulting in shortage of breath. Girls may develop breasts that are asymmetrical. Later in life, scoliotic patients develop early degenerative joint diseases and hip arthritis.

Diagnosis of scoliosis may be a spot diagnosis. However, in mild forms it may not be as visible. X-rays are required to reveal the extent to which the spine is curved. Disease progression of scoliosis can be measured by consecutive X-rays, done with measuring of the angle of curvature. Mild scoliosis has an angle below 20 degrees; moderate has between 20 and 75 degrees; severe has between 75 and 100 degrees, while the very severe has at least 100 degrees.

Treatment of scoliosis involves observation, especially for mild scoliosis as they often do not require treatment. The scoliosis will not progress once spinal bones are mature. For moderate to severe scoliosis, braces may be used to hold the back in a forced erect position until the child grows. Without a brace, the spinal position can become very deformed as the disease progresses. In very severe forms, spinal stabilization surgery may be performed, where implants or rods are used to keep the back straight. Another surgery that is often performed is spinal fusion.

Alternative methods like acupuncture, neuro-stimulation and physiotherapy have no research evidence to support their role in scoliosis treatment.

Chapter 4: Hip arthritis

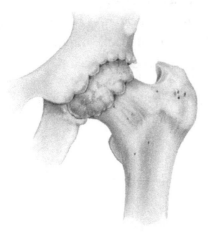

Hip arthritis is a common cause of hip pain. Arthritis of the hip is frequent in adults of +45 years of age; however, it can affect any individual at any time.

Arthritis is the inflammation of a joint, in this case of the hip. In most types of arthritis, inflammation is present but is not the main reason for which the hip joint becomes arthritic. This means that arthritis of the hip is specific to the kind of arthritis the patient has. Over 100 different types of arthritis are known, some frequently occurring like osteoarthritis, while others are very rare. One thing, however, is common in all forms of arthritis: they cause damage to the articulating cartilage of the hip joint, resulting in friction between bones.

Arthritis may occur as a complication of a condition, an example being trauma. After any injury to a joint, where the articulating cartilage is injured, or a fracture passes through a joint, 5-10 years later post-traumatic arthritis is bound to become symptomatic. Joint cartilage is very delicate. It is also irreparable when it gets injured as it does not have a repair mechanism. This is why any injury to cartilage appears to be a downhill battle with slow to fast progression of the condition. However, in children, since they are still growing, a few may be lucky enough to have their cartilage grow back as it was before, though its quality and strength will never be the same.

Hip arthritis is one common reason for inactivity in the elderly. It may exist as part of another disease condition. Autoimmune disorders like systemic lupus erythematosus and rheumatic disease are the frequently encountered. Systemic lupus erythematosus's clinical picture involves multiple joint pain due to arthritis, with or without joint effusion. A doctor's knowledge of such diseases will help in arriving at the correct diagnosis on time.

All forms of hip arthritis have arthralgia (joint pain) as the main patient complaint. Hip arthralgia is often felt during activities like walking and running. Patients of hip arthritis will have to find ways in which they can remain active, yet not inflict pain upon themselves. Without activity, the affected joint and several others become stiff and even more painful. Hip stiffness is yet another frequent finding in hip arthritis sufferers. Before patients start walking soon after waking up, they need to do some form of stretching exercises to release the joint stiffness and allow the hip to move freely. Without stretching, forced activity in a stiff hip will result in further damage such as tendon tears, muscle pull and injury to the joint capsule.

In this chapter, 5 main forms of hip arthritis are going to be discussed in detail. These include osteoarthritis, rheumatoid arthritis, septic arthritis, reactive arthritis and gout arthritis of the hip.

1) Osteoarthritis of the hip

Osteoarthritis of the hip is the second most common type after osteoarthritis of the knee. It is sometimes referred to as degenerative arthritis of the hip. Hip osteoarthritis accounts for many of the total hip replacements that are done yearly in the U.K. and the U.S. In a normal hip, the smooth articular cartilage, together with the lubricating synovial fluid provide a freely mobile joint. In hip osteoarthritis, the cartilage of the femur head and the acetabulum become rough and eroded, resulting in friction and more injury to these surfaces. When the two surfaces rub against each other, severe pain is felt by a sufferer, causing psychological stress and fear of moving the joint, thus they become very inactive. Osteoarthritis of the hip mostly occurs in a particular group of people if compared to others. This is so because of predisposing risk factors. Obesity is one such risk factor. Obese individuals develop hip arthritis early and more frequently than people of a normal weight. The hip is a weight-bearing joint. When the amount of load increases and the hip has to carry it, its wear and tear also increases. This can be compared to depreciation of a car as it is used. Age is another risk factor. Osteoarthritis is not a disease of the elderly; however, higher age groups mostly suffer from this disease. Most body tissues are made up of collagen, which is a protein substance that is abundant in the human body. With age, the collagen fibers in cartilage degenerate, resulting in loss of strength and poor nutrition of the cartilage cells (chondrocytes), making one susceptible to easy injury. Once injured, the body, in an attempt to renew itself, will form new bone. This new bone can be visualized on an X-ray as osteophytes or bony spurs. Women often suffer from osteoarthritis of the hip. This is due to low blood level hormones once menopause is reached. Osteoporosis and osteomalacia contribute to the early formation of hip arthritis.

Osteoarthritis of the hip also increases in family members of sufferers. There are many different hereditary links associated with its development. Neurological damage may result in loss of sensation at the hip, so a person will keep on walking on an injured hip without knowing. This type of joint damage is called a Charcot joint and it leads to severe damage to the hip joint. Previous injury is contributory as it causes post-traumatic hip arthritis within 10 years. Post-traumatic arthritis is one reason that hip arthritis can appear at an early age. Some concomitant diseases such as diabetes mellitus, hypertension, and sickle cell can predispose an individual to hip arthritis development.

1) Symptoms

Symptoms of hip osteoarthritis are specific to its diagnosis. Hip pain is the main complaint, and in this case it is associated with activity. As the condition progresses, the hip pain appears even at rest and it becomes sharp in character. The hip joint may be stiff and tender during a physical examination, with reduced range of movement at the hip. Reduced range of movement at the hip is a sign of impending disability. Osteoarthritis often causes a deformation in appearance of any joint. Due to the development of bony spurs and osteophytes, the hip becomes bulky and huge. A joint effusion is very common, which causes swelling at the hip and visible fluctuations as the fluid in the joint moves or is moved. In some circumstances, the osteophytes at the hip break off and become free bodies that move in the hip joint. Patients may then complain of feeling something moving inside the joint and at times catching and locking.

It is of utmost importance to understand that osteoarthritis is not a disease that is confined to the hip alone. It often affects other joints simultaneously like the joints of the spine and the hands. The fingers of an individual who suffers from osteoarthritis are thicker than usual, with a lump-like appearance at the end joints of the fingers.

2) Diagnosis

Like any other medical condition, a doctor performs a thorough physical examination. The results of this examination are then added to a clinical picture of complaints, symptoms and signs. Medical tests are then done to rule out candidate diagnosis so as to arrive to one final diagnosis. X-rays are the cheapest and most easily accessible imaging tests. It reveals osteophytes, bony spurs, reduced hip joint space, subchondral cysts and some marginal sclerosis. These often suffice to make the diagnosis of hip arthritis. Blood work is also mandatory, although most of the blood tests are non-specific. These tests include erythrocyte sedimentation rate (ESR), full blood picture (FBP) and C-reactive protein (CRP). ESR is a test that involves dropping a drop of blood into a test tube of fluid, then measuring the time it takes the drop of blood to reach the base of the test tube. In systemic conditions like cancer and tuberculosis, ESR is usually high, ranging above 60 mm/hr. In conditions like hip osteoarthritis, ESR may be normal, around 15-20 mm/hr. CRP is an early marker of inflammation. It is produced by the liver in response to stress.

3) Treatment

Hip osteoarthritis treatment has quite a number of methods to alleviate its symptoms. These methods can be conservative or surgical.

a) Conservative treatment

Pain management is the initial treatment administered to sufferers. NSAIDs like naproxen and ibuprofen are usually prescribed. However, depending on the response to pain medication, if the desired effect is not produced, other more potent drugs are substituted. Corticosteroid injections are another group of drugs often used. They are injected directly into the affected hip joint. Corticosteroid injections need to be done by someone who is used to performing such a procedure, and it requires sterile conditions. If it is performed in unsterile conditions, pathogens can be inoculated into the joint, resulting in a septic arthritis, which is more urgent than osteoarthritis. Some studies have also shown that corticosteroid injections cause erosions in the cartilage, which is known as chondrolysis. Chondrolysis on its own as an injury to a joint causes a lot of pain, so having it added to osteoarthritis worsens the disease.

Limiting the hip joint movement in a brace or splint is said to temporarily relieve pain. However, prolonged hip joint immobilization may lead to joint stiffness and muscle wasting, both of which have a poor prognostic indication to the hip joint function. Assisted mobility also helps to reduce pain by distributing the pain that a joint has to carry. Assisted walking includes crutches, walkers and wheelchairs.

Physiotherapy is a good treatment for any joint. It maintains joint function and range of motion. One does not have to perform very vigorous exercises and/or high-energy exercises, simple stretches done at home as self-care are very helpful to an ailing joint. Before any exercises are started, it is recommended to consult a physiotherapist. During the consultations, a physiotherapist has to teach you how to correctly perform particular exercises and stretches. If exercises are done in a wrong way, they can lead to further damage to the joint and/or imbalance, e.g. unbalanced muscle group strength.

Home remedies include hot and cold therapies. This treatment modality is specific to an individual; some people respond well when cold is applied to the joint, while others respond to heat. It's basically trying this and that to find out what best suits you. Cold therapy involves wrapping some ice cubes in a towel, and then applying it to the joint for 15-20 minutes. Never apply ice blocks directly to skin as it causes a thermal burn. Substitutes to ice blocks can be used, like disposable ice packs. A disposable ice pack is made up of a chemical that is placed in a plastic wrap. Inside this liquid is another plastic with crystals of another chemical component. To make the disposable ice pack cold, one has to squeeze the plastic inside the liquid chemical to release the crystals into the liquid. Then shake for a chemical reaction to take place between the chemical liquid and the crystals. This reaction gives adequate cold to treat a joint for about 10 minutes. Once used, the chemicals are used up and are not reusable. In heat therapy, warm water is placed in a bucket. Then a towel is soaked in the water for a few minutes. The excess water is squeezed out, and the warm towel is applied on the joint. Hot therapy to the hip can also be performed by sitting in a dish of warm water, or by soaking oneself in a bathtub of warm water. Hot or cold therapy can be repeated twice or thrice daily.

Lifestyle changes are usually helpful in hip osteoarthritis treatment. Losing weight will help reduce the weight that the ill hip has to carry. Eating healthily will help in tissue repair and healing. Foods that have calcium and anti-inflammatory effects are recommended, like milk, fish, omega-3 and walnuts. Natural foods do not only help in weight loss, but they have been reported by some sufferers to reduce pain. A natural diet consist of unprocessed foods, in their raw state, e.g. butternut squash, lentils, and leafy vegetables like spinach.

Alternative treatment methods for osteoarthritis include ultrasound therapy, shockwave therapy and acupuncture. However, these methods have not been thoroughly researched as to their actual role in treatment of osteoarthritis of the hip.

b) Surgical treatment

When conservative measures do not yield the desired effects, surgery is the next option. However, surgery may be indicated from the start of certain conditions. Surgery of the hip can be performed as an open or "key hole" surgery. Due to cosmetic problems after an open surgery, most patients tend to prefer "key hole" surgery, which is also known as arthroscopy. In arthroscopy, a surgeon makes an incision of about 0.5-1cm, and then introduces a fiber-optic tubing that has a camera at the end for visualization. During an arthroscopy, a surgeon can clean the hip joint of debris and growths, and labral and cartilage tears can be repaired. For individuals who have some misalignment at the hip, coxa vara or coxa valgus, a corrective osteotomy can be performed. If the hip joint surfaces have severely eroded, a total hip replacement can be done.

Hip replacement surgery can be partial or total. It is known as arthroplasty. Hip arthroplasty is performed on failed hip joints that cannot be treated by conservative means. In these cases, the patient's main complaint will be pain. Hip arthroplasty consists of two components: the acetabular component and the femur component. The acetabular component can be made from metal or polyethylene. This acetabulum can be a single piece or it can be modular. A modular acetabular component consists of an outer cup and an inner cup. This design is intended to enhance function of the hip by making movement smooth and frictionless. When the acetabulum is fixed, it can be held in place by screws or bone cement.

The femur component consists of a stalk and the head. Many brands are available on the market, and the most common are titanium, stainless steel, and combinations of different alloys, including chromium. The bone marrow of the femur is removed proximally to create room for insertion of the stalk. The femur component can be held in place by bone cement, or by design.

A major complication of hip arthroplasty is infection. Once an implant is infected, treatment measures change, since they have to be removed. The infection is then treated with the application of local antibiotic beads and joint debridement. Only after the infection has cleared, another attempt at hip arthroplasty can be made. However, a once-infected joint has a greater chance of being re-infected.

In developing countries where hip replacement equipment or implants may not be readily available, they perform an operation called girdlestone. Girdlestone is when the femur head is removed, and the space is left without any fixations or artificial head application. The patient is then put on skeletal traction to lengthen the limb while fibrous tissue develops to fill in the gap that remains after the femur head is removed. After three weeks on skeletal traction, the patient is then taught by the physiotherapist how to walk. Most patients will develop a limp, as the operated leg will be about 2-3cm shorter than the other. This complication can be treated by a shoe raise of 2-3cm. The last option to relieve pain is a hip arthrodesis or hip fusion. An arthrodesis would fuse the femur head to the acetabulum. This means that the joint will not be functional to bend or straighten. It will remain straight at all times, but pain-free.

2) Rheumatoid arthritis of the hip

Rheumatoid arthritis (RA) of the hip is the second most prevalent arthritis of the hip. RA is a systemic immunological disease, which arises after a trigger factor initiates an immunological response to self. In the human body, immunity protects the body against diseases. However, in RA, the antibodies that are meant to attack foreign organisms attack the normal tissues of the joint. It is very rare to find RA localized only to the hip joint. It tends to affect multiple joints at once, and other body tissues such as tendons and ligaments. RA usually affects symmetrical joints of the body and weight-bearing joints.

Being a woman and being overweight predisposes an individual to the development of RA. The chances also increase when a relative or a family member suffers from the disease. RA includes chronic inflammation of the hip. This means that signs of acute inflammation like heat, swelling and tenderness may not be as obvious.

RA diagnosis is often made when a patient experiences symptoms such as pain and fatigue. RA of the hip affects anyone at any age, although individuals between 40-60, especially women, are most commonly affected. More than 70% of RA cases are in females. RA of any joint, including the hip, has 4 stages of development.

Stage 1: Individuals at this stage are unaware that they have the disease. Generally patients will not have complaints or symptoms. However, this is the stage at which the immune system begins to attack its own tissue cells.

Stage 2: This stage marks the development and persistence of inflammation. The hip joint becomes swollen, tender, and painful. Additionally, overgrowth of joint tissues such as the joint capsule, and over-production of synovial fluid are also present during this stage. The fluctuation test of the hip may be positive. The main complaint of sufferers is pain, which is associated with joint swelling due to new blood vessels that form and congest the joint.

Stage 3: Joint injury becomes more evident. This is due to the fact that inflammation persists in the hip joint. Waste substances and enzymes found in the joint due to chronic inflammation erode the cartilage of articular surfaces. The severity of pain increases, most patients report gritting sounds and free particles that move within the hip joint. Bone moves against bone, causing severe pain.

Stage 4: This stage marks a worsening condition at the hip joint, which by now is irreversible; the joint is disfigured. Patients at this stage may benefit from a total hip replacement.

1) Risk factors

RA is likely to affect individuals that are genetically predisposed to the disease. A healthy person following a healthy lifestyle may develop RA because, genetically, they are at risk of developing the disease. Individuals that have a close relative who suffers from RA have a higher risk of developing the disease over time. Studies show that people with the human leukocytic antigen (HLA-DR4) are naturally at risk of developing RA.

Women over 40 years old are also at high risk of developing RA. This is likely due to the fact that at this age hormones like estrogen and progesterone become low in the blood as menopause sets in. Postmenopausal women are at an even greater risk of developing RA. Some systemic diseases that have immunological pathogenesis are linked to RA development. These diseases include systemic lupus erythematosus and scleroderma. Highly stressed individuals are also more likely to develop RA symptoms than happier individuals. Stress is related to alcohol use and cigarette smoking; both habits increase the chance of developing RA. Individuals that have RF in their blood, and a high ESR or CRP, have a risk of developing RA at some point in their lives.

2) Symptoms

A doctor may diagnose RA after a thorough physical examination and medical tests. Some of its symptoms are pain, swelling of the joint, and tenderness. Morning stiffness, which lasts for 30-45 minutes is a particularly common symptom of RA. This morning stiffness goes away once one does some stretches and exercises of the joint. RA symptoms appear as flare-ups—periodically, with remissions. A remission is a time during which an individual who has been diagnosed with RA has no symptoms or pain. As the disease progresses, flare-ups become increasingly frequent and remissions become increasingly short lived, until eventually symptoms are constant; symptoms can become so frequent that they disrupt a patient's sleep.

RA affects the stabilizing components of the hip, especially the ligaments, loosening them. This laxity causes instability within the joint, making it susceptible to injury like subluxation, dislocation, and fracture.

Patients with RA tend to have a limping gait, due to the body modifying the normal gait to decrease the weight bearing on the affected hip. Because RA is a systemic disease, what many know as rheumatism, general body symptoms such as fatigue, muscle aches and sweating may be present. RA affects other body organs such that the appearance of certain signs in other body tissues may lead a doctor to suspect RA. These conditions include vasculitis, inflammation of the eyes, nodules under the skin, and nerve compression syndromes like carpal tunnel and tarsal tunnel.

3) Diagnosis

There are 2 types of RA- one with slow and steady progression, known as benign RA, and one that is very aggressive. Clinically, a doctor suspects RA when one has morning stiffness for more than 30 minutes in the joints of the hands and other symmetrical joints, nodules under the skin, swollen or deformed fingers and toes, deviations of the joints, especially the wrists, and pain of symmetrical joints.

The patient's life history is important, and the results of tests like ESR and CRP may be high, although not always. FBP shows signs of chronic inflammation like lymphocytosis. RF may be positive, however the diagnosis of RA is still possible if RF is negative. Plain joint X-rays may show changes in hip arthritis, reduced joint space, soft tissue swelling, or they may appear normal. A reliable method for diagnosing RA is checking synovial fluid aspirate for increased cells and debris, as markers of chronic inflammation.

Other types of hip arthritis, such as osteoarthritis, a gouty hip, post-traumatic arthritis and reactive arthritis should be eliminated before diagnosing RA.

4) Treatment

The first therapy that a sufferer can initiate at home is the RICE method. The RICE method is used to alleviate pain in most conditions resulting from inflammation. The method encourages individuals to Rest, Ice, Compress, and Elevate. To rest a limb, one should temporarily avoid using it. In this case, one should avoid walking in order to rest the hip joint. Ice means cooling off an inflamed joint by applying ice wrapped in a towel, artificial cooling substances, or freeze-wraps. Compression requires one to apply a brace or crepe bandage as a way to alleviate pain. The limb is then propped up on a pile of pillows to aid drainage of the lymphatic system from the limb back to the heart and reduce swelling.

NSAIDs are effective for relief of pain caused by RA. However, disease modifying anti-rheumatic drugs (DMARDs) such as methotrexate and sulfasalazine are the best choice. As always, your doctor will have to prescribe these medications. Some recent DMARDs consist of biological medicines such as Enbrel, which may have some side effects that a patient should be well aware of before the drugs can be used.

Corticosteroid injections, gold injections, and hyaluronic acid injections are available on the market as temporary pain relievers. Physical therapy is necessary to preserve joint function. Alternative methods including acupuncture, shock-wave therapy, and ultrasound treatment require further research as to their role in the pain relief of RA.

Some patients apply arthritic creams daily on the affected hip. Some creams available are Zostrix arthritis cream, Bengay, Tiger Balm, Icy Hot, and Osmoflex. Most of these soothing creams have menthol as the main ingredient. Some topical gels include Fastumgel and Capzasin P. For more information, see www.walgreens.com and www.webmd.com.

Surgery for RA is not always a last resort. Synovectomy, a procedure that can be done to debride a hypertrophic synovial membrane, can be performed by arthroscopy. When the joint structure is beyond repair and is severely deformed, a hip replacement can be done.

Modifying equipment around the house is of great benefit to RA sufferers. Dressing aids including a shoe horn with a long handle, shoe horn reacher, a sock aid, and arthritic hip kits help sufferers dress easily. For more information, visit www.arthtritissupplies.com.

3) A gouty hip

Gout arthritis (GA) is a common disease that is more common in males younger than 65 than in females. Additionally, African-Americans are commonly affected. Gout will affect 10 to 20 people out of every 1,000. In America, about 1 million people are diagnosed with GA every year.

GA of the hip is rare;the disease usually affects the big toes, knees, elbows and wrists. Since GA is a systemic condition, many joints are often affected simultaneously.

GA is a disease caused by the development of crystals within joints. These monosodium urate crystals form lumps and stones within the joint.

When humans eat food, waste products exit the body through urine, sweat, and feces. Protein-rich substances such as meat produce purines from deoxyribonucleic acid (DNA) and ribonucleic acid (RNA) compounds found in its tissue cells. These purines are broken down to produce uric acid, which is excreted in urine. Abundant uric acid production is associated with GA. Overproduction of uric acid is due to overeating purine-containing foods such red meat and seafood. The uric acid levels in the blood increase significantly, known as hyperuricemia. Hyperuricemia may be present in an individual that has not yet been diagnosed with GA but is an early presentation of GA. Because of high levels of uric acid in the blood, the body attempts to maintain the blood's acidity and balance by removing excess uric acid. This uric acid accumulates in joints and soft tissues of the body. In joints, the uric acid crystallizes to form monosodium urate crystals. The presence of these crystals causes joint inflammation and the development of arthritis.

Gout arthritis development occurs in 4 stages:

Stage 1- An individual experiences no signs and symptoms of GA, although blood tests may show hyperuricemia.

Stage 2- The monosodium urate crystals begin to accumulate in the joint, triggering inflammation. Symptoms of inflammation become evident; and the individual tends to visit their GP with complains of pain, redness, swelling, and heat. Gout is often marked as podagra at this stage—symptoms appear on the big toe. Blood tests for uric acid may show normal levels, because the excess uric acid is in joints and tissues rather than the blood.

Stage 3- The disease progresses as urate crystals continue to accumulate within the joint. This results in a chronic inflammation, which leads to cartilage abrasion and injury. The disease appears as flare-ups and remissions. A flare-up occurs when the disease is visibly active. The joint is swollen, red, hot, and very painful. RA also has flare-ups and remissions in its course; the two types of arthritis require correct differentiation from one another.

Stage 4- GA is now clinically diagnosed with the help of a patient's history. Crystals that accumulate in the joint form lumps called tophi. Tophi often grow in areas where there is a lot of pressure, such as the elbows and knees. These are cosmetically irritating to many sufferers and many may opt for surgery to remove them.

1) Risk factors

Males are 4 times more likely than women to develop gout in their lifetime. Gout most commonly affects individuals between 40-50 years of age. People who suffer from diseases that may result in hyperuricemia, like kidney disease and metabolic states, also have an increased risk of developing GA. Medications such as diuretics are known to increase the risk of GA. Dietary risks leading to GA involve eating a high purine content diet, such as one rich in game meat. However, hereditary risks are also a contributing factor to the development of GA, even in individuals without any of the other risks.

2) Signs and symptoms

Symptoms appear and disappear, in flare-ups and remissions. During a flare-up, the joint can become very swollen, red, and hot within 24 hours. A single joint is often affected, although multiple joints can be affected because of GA's systemic pathogenesis. The skin above the joint may be itchy, and the skin may begin peeling off. Pain often occurs at night. Hyperuricemia may be present. Even before a GA diagnosis, an experienced physician will not miss gout tophi.

3) Diagnosis

A GA diagnosis is similar to most medical conditions. It requires a thorough review of the patient's symptoms. A doctor will ask for a complete patient history, and then perform a physical examination. These procedures should be sufficient for a diagnosis. In other cases, blood tests may be performed including tests of uric acid levels of blood, ESR, CRP, and FBP. X-rays may show tophi, but not always. General signs of arthritis like reduced joint space or calcification of tendons will be taken into account.

However, the gold standard for GA diagnosis is examination of a joint aspirate under the microscope, where crystals are seen.

4) Treatment

The short term goal of GA treatment is to eliminate pain, while the long-term goal is to reduce the production of uric acid. The RICE method can be used in flare-ups. Cooling the joint gives some relief since a gouty joint is hot and red when it's active. NSAIDs like Naproxen and Ibuprofen can be taken as pain management medications. For GA, corticosteroids can be taken as tablets or shots directly into the joint. They too help eliminate inflammation, therefore pain. They are medications that can be dangerous if used improperly, hence they require your GP's prescription. Drugs like Colchicine and Allopurinol prevent overproduction of uric acid. Their use during flare-ups is controversial because they have been shown to worsen symptoms. Dietary manipulation is another way to prevent uric acid overproduction. A vegan diet is ideal, but not a must. If meat must be consumed, it should be taken in small portions, preferably the white meat. Splinting the joint with a brace during a flare-up has been reported by some sufferers to be helpful. A brace offloads some weight on a joint. Continuing to move the affected joint by stretching and exercise, as in physical therapy, maintains joint function. Without physical therapy, a gouty joint can become stiff and contracted permanently. A surgical washout can also be performed in severe conditions that have a lot of floating crystals in the joint. Tophi can be surgically removed, and the joint debridged.

4) Others

GA, OA and RA are not the only forms of arthritis that can affect the hip. In individuals that had an injury to the hip in the previous years, pain at the hip may be post-traumatic arthritis. Post-traumatic arthritis occurs within 5-10 years after injury to the hip, especially fractures that extend within the joint. On X-rays, post-traumatic arthritis appears like osteoarthritis, only that the joint is often more severely damaged than an osteoarthritis that has developed by itself. In the lifetime of any human, hip arthritis is bound to develop at some point; however, the speed of its development is faster in a previously injured hip. Post-traumatic arthritis is one of the reasons that a young individual can develop early hip arthritis.

Injuries to the hip may occur due to falls, especially in the elderly, motor traffic accidents, gunshot injury and spontaneous hip injuries. These injuries may be open or closed. An open hip injury will further increase the risk of developing yet a different type of arthritis, septic arthritis. Septic arthritis occurs when disease causing pathogens make their way into the joint. In the majority of cases, it is due to an open injury. However, pathogens can be brought to the hip joint via blood from other sites e.g. a urinary tract infection. Staphylococcus aureus is the pathogen that is often isolated during pus cultures in the laboratory.

The main goals of treating hip arthritis are to alleviate pain, to stop or reduce the speed of disease progression, and to maintain hip function. It is very unfortunate that hip arthritis has no cure, but with the correct measures, sufferers can have a comfortable, active life.

Chapter 5: Hip joint physiotherapy

Exercise is good for many body organs; the heart, the lungs and the brain among others. People who suffer from hip arthritis avoid activities that aggravate pain; this is innate behavior in every human being in order to prevent harm. However, when arthritic hips are left immobile for a long time, they become stiff and lose the ability to move, which is known as ankylosis. Exercises are therefore good for arthritic hips, since they are prophylaxis to a worsening joint condition. For clarity, I have to mention that exercises do not cure an arthritic hip, but simply improve the condition. Exercises for the hip do not have to be vigorous; simple stretches like a twenty-minute walk can do much for a joint.

Joint exercises fall under physiotherapy. Physiotherapy is a branch of medicine that uses exercise to improve chronic conditions like arthritis, stroke, scoliosis and trauma. Physiotherapy does not deal only with exercise; it offers other pain-relieving treatment modalities, like ultrasound therapy and shockwave therapy. A professional who performs physiotherapy is called a physiotherapist. Like any medical professional, a physiotherapist also gets registered and certified by the board of physiotherapists. Physiotherapists are available in most trauma or orthopedic centers, in sports centers, NHS hospitals and community support centers. One can locate a physiotherapist in any region in the UK or US by "Googling" a post code or area code on Google Maps.

This chapter covers some of the exercises that you can do safely at home, although a go ahead is required from your GP beforehand. It is also a good idea to have a physiotherapist initially show you how to correctly do these exercises, after which you can continue on your own at home. Improper exercise techniques may further damage the affected hip joint and/or cause a different problem in other body parts.

1) Tips for good exercises

- ❖ Take a warm shower or sit in a warm whirlpool before exercising.

- ❖ Warm up first before any activity.

- ❖ Gear up appropriately for exercise. Loose clothes are good, with a light material which dries off quickly when you sweat. Shoes with good arch support, shock absorbers and non-slip technology are recommended.

- ❖ During the exercise, be slow and careful, there is no hurry.

- ❖ Take short breaks in between exercise routines.

- ❖ Remember to breathe adequately.

- ❖ Rehydrate as often as possible.

- ❖ Be gentle with tender and swollen joints.

- ❖ Even with a flare-up, do some simple stretches to maintain joint movement.

- ❖ Count each step loudly; it helps with your breathing and concentration.

- ❖ Overall, do not over-exert a joint that is having a flare-up.

- ❖ Knowing when to stop is essential and lifesaving. Stop immediately if you feel sudden, sharp pain, when you feel nauseous or dizzy, when your chest becomes tight with breathing difficulties or when you have heart palpitations and severe fatigue.

❖ Exercise routines take a while before you can see results. Therefore, discipline and courage is needed to stick to the exercise routine.

❖ Invite a friend or family member to join your routines. An exercise companion can be encouraging and supportive when you feel down.

❖ Spice up your daily routines by doing exercises that you enjoy. Playing music that you like while you exercise can be fun too.

❖ Move your exercise to a different level as your joints improve. For example, move from simple stretching routines to strengthening exercises.

❖ Consult your GP when you feel any one of the following: increased pain, persistent body fatigue, reduced joint range of motion and muscle weakness or paralysis.

2) Hip exercises

Below are some exercise routines that you can try. Always consult your doctor first before doing exercises as I do not know your medical history.

A) Walking, cycling and swimming

These activities should be done to a level that you can tolerate. Do not overdo it. Walking may be painful if you use an uneven or rocky path. At first, try a smooth pavement, with little to no incline, and then intensify the exercise as you improve. A stationary bike can also be used for hip exercises. As you move your legs in circles, a recumbent bike increases the angle between the thigh and the hip, thus improving the range of motion of the joint. When walking or cycling is too painful to be included in your daily routine, swimming may be the best option for you. Water helps your joints support your weight, and by doing so, enhances joint mobility.

B) Leg swings

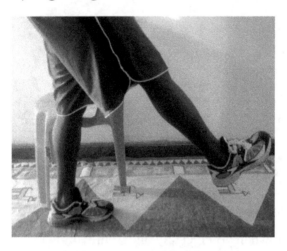

1) Hold the edge of the table for support.

2) Keeping your body in a straight position, swing your right leg outwards and inwards 10 times at a moderate speed.

3) Repeat with your left leg.

4) This exercise may be done 3-4 times a day.

C) Leg extensions

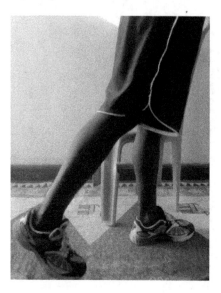

1) Hold the edge of the table for support, with your body in an erect position.

2) Stretch your right leg backwards as far as you can.

3) Hold the position for 6 seconds.

4) Release the hold and return your leg to a neutral position.

5) Repeat the same movement using your left leg.

6) This stretch can be performed 3-4 times every day.

D) Straight leg lifting

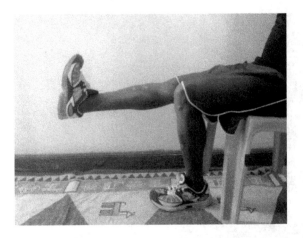

1) Sit on a chair with your legs together and feet flat on the floor.

2) Raise one leg straight up in front of you.

3) Hold the position for 5 seconds.

4) Release and bring the leg back to its neutral position.

5) Repeat with the other leg.

6) This exercise can be done 4-5 times on each leg.

E) Pelvic thrusts

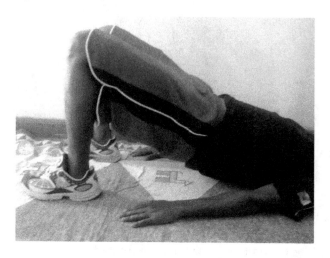

1) Lie on the floor on your back with your knees bent. Make sure that your feet are flat on the floor.

2) Thrust only your pelvis up, lifting your buttocks off the ground.

3) Hold the position for 6 seconds, and then release your buttocks back onto the floor.

4) Repeat this routine 4-5 times.

Tip

Keep your hands off the ground. You can rest them on your abdomen.

F) Angry cat stretch

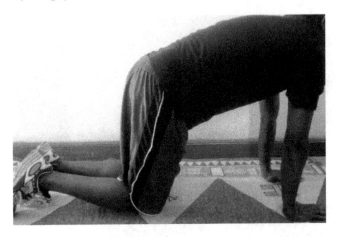

1) Kneel down on the ground on your knees and hands.

2) Arch your back up like an angry cat.

3) Hold the position for 6 seconds.

4) Release and repeat the exercise 5 times.

Tips

- If your hip pain is a result of a herniated disc and/or any other back problem, you should avoid this exercise.

- Hip joints function together with other joints like the back and knees. Exercising these other joints together with your hips will help improve your overall condition. Besides, most hip arthritis affects other joints of the body as well; degenerative joint disease of the spine is one of the frequently occurring conditions.

G) Single knee pull

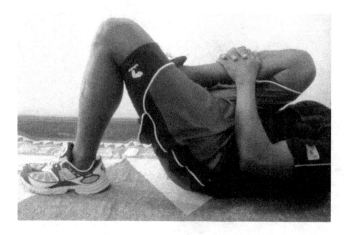

1) Lie on your back with both your knees bent, keeping your feet flat on the floor.

2) Bring one knee up against your stomach.

3) Pull the knee against your stomach using both your hands until you feel a stretch in your buttock.

4) Hold the position for 6 seconds.

5) Release and repeat using the other knee to make one cycle.

6) Rest for a few seconds, and then repeat 3 more cycles.

H) Double knee pull

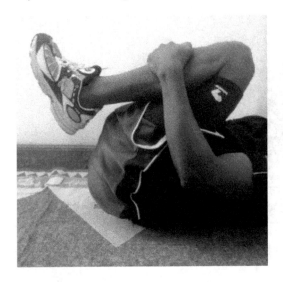

1) Lie on your back with both your knees bent, keeping your feet flat on the ground.

2) Bring both your knees up against your abdomen.

3) Using your hands, fix your raised knees against your stomach.

4) Slightly raise your head up, moving your chin to touch your knees.

5) Hold the position for 5 seconds.

6) Release and rest for a few seconds, and repeat 5-6 times.

I) Hip kicks

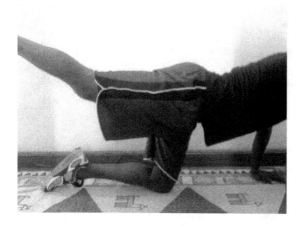

1) Kneel down on your knees and hands.

2) Keeping your back straight, carefully raise one leg straight behind you.

3) Hold the outstretched leg position for 6 seconds, and then return it to the starting position.

4) Do the same with the other leg.

5) Repeat the routine 4-5 times on each leg.

Tips

- Patients with hip pain due to back problems should not do this exercise.

- As your hip joint's mobility improves with exercise, the "hip kick" routine can be intensified by tying small weights at the ankle.

J) Standing heel raise

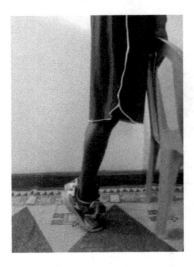

1) Stand behind a chair, holding the backrest for support.

2) Slowly raise your heels up so you're standing on tiptoes.

3) Hold the position for 6 seconds, and then release.

4) Repeat the raise and release movement 10 times.

Tip

- This exercise strengthens hip and cuff muscles.

- It also improves balance.

K) Heel slides

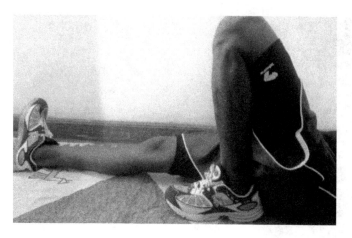

1) Lie on the floor on your back.

2) Stretch both your legs straight in front of you, placing them together.

3) Keeping your heels flat on the floor, slide your left heel upwards towards your buttock as far as you can, bending your knee and hip in the process.

3) Hold the position for 6 seconds.

4) Slowly release to starting position.

5) Repeat the same procedure with your other leg.

6) Repeat 10-20 times, 3 times daily.

Tip

This exercise is good when it is done early in the morning to loosen morning joint stiffness.

L) Single leg stand

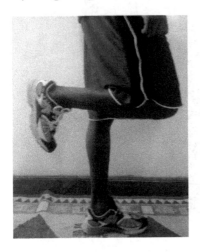

1) Stand in an erect position with your feet together.

2) Lift your better leg up so you're standing on the arthritic leg for as long as you can tolerate.

3) Release the hold, and rest for a few seconds.

4) Repeat again 3-4 times.

Tip

Throw and catch a ball while you stand on the arthritic leg. This will further strengthen your balance and intensify the routine.

M) Side-lying leg lift

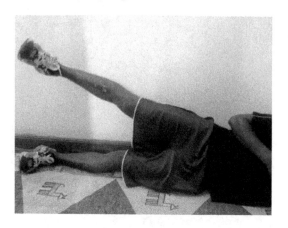

1) Lie on your side on the floor, supporting the head with the elbow.

2) Slowly raise the top leg up and down, keeping it in a straight position.

3) Repeat 10 times, and then roll over to switch leg positions and repeat the exercise.

Tip

This exercise can be intensified by holding a small weight on top of the thigh as you raise your leg up and down.

N) Hamstring wall stretch

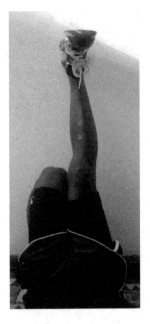

1) Lie on your back, with your buttocks close to a wall and your knees bent.

2) Raise one leg up against the wall for 20 seconds.

3) Bring the raised leg down into its initial bent position, and prop the other leg up against the wall.

4) Repeat the routine 4-5 times.

O) Ilio-tibial band stretch

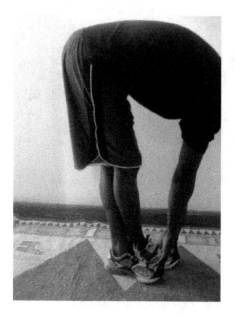

1) Stand in an upright position.

2) Cross your legs over each other.

3) Bend over to touch your toes, keeping your legs straight and in a crossed-over position.

4) Hold the position for 20 seconds, and come back up.

5) Repeat the exercise 5 times.

P) Iliopsoas muscle stretch

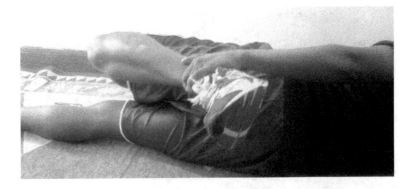

1) Lie on your side with both your legs in a straight position.

2) Grab the ankle of the uppermost leg and pull it backwards, bending the knee as far as you can.

3) Hold the position for 20 seconds, then release and rest for 5 seconds.

4) Repeat the process again on the other side.

Q) Gluteus stretch

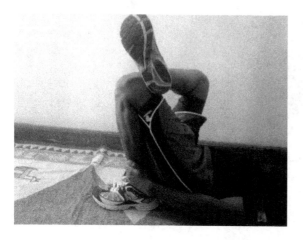

1) Lie on the floor on your back with both knees bent.

2) Raise the ankle of one leg to sit on the knee of the other leg in a figure 4 position.

3) Pull the bottom thigh towards you as far as you can to stretch both the gluteal region of the lower thigh and the hip of the leg on top.

4) Hold the position for 20 seconds, then release and switch the limb position.

R) Adductor stretch

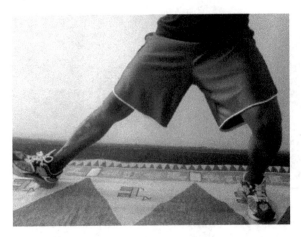

1) Stand up straight with your feet apart.

2) Bend one knee while the other stays straight.

3) Lower yourself down as far as possible to feel a stretch in the inner thigh of the straight leg and the groin of the other.

4) Hold the position for 20 seconds and come back up.

5) Rest for 5 seconds and repeat the routine again.

S) Cross-leg side lift

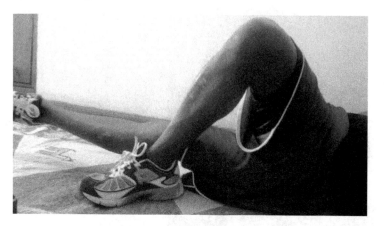

1) Lie on your side with your legs in a straight position and support the head with the elbow.

2) Cross the top leg over the bottom one to form the figure 4.

3) Raise the straight leg (the one below) slowly up and down.

4) Repeat the up-down movement 10 times and switch leg positions.

T) Hip external rotation

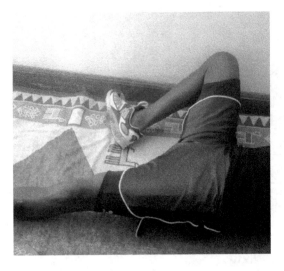

1) Lie on your back with one knee bent and the other straight.

2) Take the bent knee to the side as far as you can to stretch the hip of the same side.

3) Hold the position for 5 seconds and move the knee inwards.

4) Repeat in and out knee movements 10 times, and then switch legs.

U) Pelvis rocking

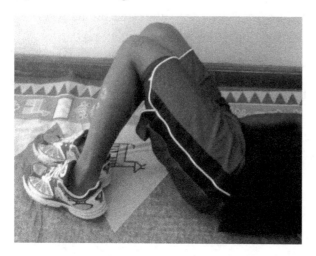

1) Lie on your back with both your knees bent.

2) Move both your knees from side to side like you are rocking while maintaining the upper body in a fixed position against the floor.

3) Rock as many times as you can.

3) Pet arthritis therapy

Dogs and cats also require exercises and other treatments when they become arthritic. Here are some therapies that one can consider:

a) Massage - Start by lightly stroking the area that you want to massage. This helps the local blood circulation. After a few minutes of light-pressure strokes, gently knead the muscles in a circular motion. Do not perform massage directly over an arthritic joint, but rather the muscles around it.

b) Hot and cold therapy can also be safely performed on your pet. This relieves pain, especially when performed on swollen, tender joints.

c) Medications like Etogesic and Rimadyl are anti-inflammatory drugs that can be given to your pet for pain relief. However, a consultation with your vet for a prescription is required.

d) Exercises - Taking your pet for a slow, 10-minute walk, making sure that the road is level, can be beneficial. Swimming for 15-20 minutes is also a perfect exercise for your dog's arthritic joints.

e) Lifestyle changes - Soft bedding offers good support for your arthritic pet. Adequate cushioning is necessary to reduce pain. Keep things in safe areas in the house. A lot of obstacles can be difficult for your pet to go around, e.g. chairs and other furniture. If your house has stairs, consider setting a ramp for your arthritic pet. Slippery floors can be dangerous for a pet with painful joints to navigate, so rugs and carpets are excellent substitutes for laminated and tiled floors.

f) Weight loss - Controlling your pet's weight will help with reducing pain; hence, weight loss programs and exercise routines should be highly prioritized. Diets like Purina, with enough amounts of substitute nutrients such as Omega 3 fatty acids, chondroitine sulphate and glucoseamine, may be helpful.

g) Family support

Family support is a crucial mental therapy. Your pet has to feel your love and support. This includes some peace and quiet when it is required, especially when children always want to play with the dog outside. Playtime can be distressing for an arthritic pet. Though playing outside can be a great exercise routine for a pet, it should be restricted. Some games that can be fun are fetch, hide and seek and soccer. Family support also includes grooming. Arthritic pets tend to reduce their grooming, especially in areas that are painful to reach. Bathing, blow drying and trimming fur should be a weekly routine.

h) Others - Low-level laser therapy, aquatic therapy, acupuncture and Adequan injections may be considered too.

Tips:

- Be reasonable—walks should be short and slow. A 10-minute walk is more tolerable than a 10-mile hike.

- Be rate-conscious—start slow and pick up tempo with time.

- Be regular—exercise must be done on a daily basis, just like your pet's meals.

- Make it fun.

- Join other pet owners with their pets, or invite your friend's or neighbor's pet.

- Do activities that both you and your pet can perform with no difficulties.

Chapter 6: Supportive treatment for hip arthritis

Supportive treatment for hip arthritis involves a lifestyle change. Lifestyle changes in this context are related to the way in which an individual with hip arthritis lives their day-to-day life. Movements that involve shaking the affected joints vigorously, e.g. vibrations, should be avoided since they increase trauma to the hip. Therefore, individuals with occupations that increase repetitive, stressful hip movements should find a way to reduce this trauma. Work can be substituted for something light, or the work area can be adjusted. The use of mechanical aids like splints or braces, shoe inserts and orthopedic shoes may help in improving the joint. Weight loss, if needed, has been proven by many studies to reduce arthritic hip pain. Diet manipulations, such as eating foods that are rich in Omega 3 fatty acids, fruits, vegetables and whole grains, can be of great benefit. Eliminating some activities that you like may be difficult; however, if they worsen joint wearing and tearing, they should be avoided. Meditation and yoga can complement medical management plans for chronic pain and the stress associated with it.

In the UK, 8.5 million people currently suffer from arthritis of the hip, knee and hands. In 20 years, the figure is estimated to rise to 17 million. Lifestyle changes are another way to tackle chronic pain that results from hip arthritis. This chapter discusses suggestions and recommendations for some changes that can be of help in day-to-day living.

1) Best mattresses

Patients have reported experiencing increased comfort with waterbeds. However, waterbed sheets are not everyone's favorite, and they are hard to find. A great selection of mattresses may seem good at the start, but a mould problem will soon get on your nerves. Getting a good mattress for hip arthritis can be very challenging, since price considerations also play a role in the final decision. Unfortunately, mattresses that actually work best for individuals with hip arthritis are a bit expensive. So, before one spends a fortune, they ought to be sure that the mattress will work as it should. Mattresses may work well for one individual, but may not work as effectively for another. Finding one specifically suited to your needs is the greatest challenge.

Some sufferers use 100% latex foam mattresses. This mattress should be tried only if you are not allergic to latex. Talalay latex is one type that can be tried. Customize a latex mattress with a local dealer as to the number of layers you want and the size. Already-made mattresses can be expensive; however, one can reduce the prize by making their own. Buy separate latex mattresses and stack them up to form a mattress. One can also buy a cover with a zipper so the self-made mattress can be contained.

Some sufferers have had relief with a 4-inch memory foam topper. This can be purchased from Ebay or Brookstone. However, the so-called viscous foam is uncomfortably hot for some people.

Other individuals add a featherbed on top of other mattresses. Feathers can evoke allergic reactions, especially allergic rhinitis. Use them only when you do not react to such a mattress.

The Arthritic Foundation recommends Tempurpedic. Some sufferers say that Tempurpedic conforms around you so that you feel like you are in a hammock when you sleep on it, while others enjoy its comfort and can actually experience a good night's sleep on it.

Mattresses with odors can also affect your sleep pattern. The Nature's Rest mattress does not smell or sink like Tempurpedic. Another good mattress that one can try is Nova-foam.

These are a few mattresses that some sufferers have found helpful for their arthritic hips and back. Mattresses can be chosen based on body weight. A firmer mattress is necessary for someone with more weight. The way in which an individual sleeps can also be used to find a suitable mattress. Side sleepers require a medium-firm to firm mattress, while a back sleeper needs a traditional, firm bed.

Tips

❖ Allow plenty of shopping time

❖ Buy your mattress during the summer sales period

❖ Consider return policies before a purchase. Many companies offer a 30-day trial, so if for whatever reason your mattress is not what you want after a week, you should be able to return it for another.

❖ Some companies that advertise returns charge a large restocking fee, so one has to watch out for this.

❖ Buying a mattress is like buying a car, do not pay retail price.

❖ If you have arthritis on one hip, sleep on the normal hip.

❖ Sleep with a pillow between your legs.

❖ Back sleepers can put a small pillow under their knees; it helps to keep the back in a normal, unstrained position.

❖ If one suffers from sleep apnea, sleeping on the side reduces back pressure and snoring.

2) Best pillows

Insomnia can also develop due to incorrect positioning of the head during sleep. Too soft or too hard of a pillow can strain your neck. A good pillow improves the quality of sleep; however, it can be hard to come by. An improper pillow can cause headaches, arm numbness, neck and shoulder pain, and even trigger symptoms of some conditions that otherwise wouldn't surface. Also, a pillow needs to be changed every 12 - 18 months for a healthy lifestyle. An old pillow often has mould, fungus and flaked-off skin cells. These can be triggers for allergic reactions.

For anyone to find a good pillow, they must define what type of sleeper they are first. A stomach sleeper will find comfort in a flat and thin-cushioned pillow (see www.selectcomfort.com). Synthetic materials like Land's End essential Pure loft are good substitutes for feathered pillows for an allergic sleeper. Back sleepers need a pillow that can support their head adequately, especially ones with a depression in the middle. Plumped-up pillows may be perfect for side sleepers.

Tips for choosing a good pillow

❖ Choose a pillow with a good and solid feeling. A pillow with loose foam is bound to break down after a few days of use. Besides, squishing a pillow into shape all the time is annoying.

❖ If you choose a feathered pillow, get one with polyester wrapping around the feathers to prevent them from getting out.

❖ If one prefers feathers, get hypoallergenic goose down.

❖ Large pillows are better as they support your head, neck and shoulders more effectively.

❖ Good pillows are often pricey, so set a budget before setting out to look for one.

❖ A good pillow keeps your spine in natural alignment.

❖ A good pillow is often 4-6 inches in height.

❖ The texture of a pillow improves comfort. One can get a soft and smooth pillow like cotton, or a warm flannel material. The pillow material may be rough, but one can get a good pillow cover to make it comfortable.

❖ Consider your partner's sleeping position too before buying new pillows.

❖ Shake and fluff out your pillow every day.

❖ A machine-washable pillow can be very handy, since it is easy to keep it clean.

3) Best shoes

Hip arthritis is a broad disease. As we understand, there are many forms of hip arthritis. A good shoe for an arthritic hip depends on the type of arthritis. People who have rheumatoid arthritis often have associated edema on the feet and flat feet. A good shoe for such an individual is one that caters to all these pathologies. A deep shoe with a removable, supportive insole is preferred. The shoe has to have a strap, since rheumatoid arthritis symptoms in the hands do not favor lace-up shoes. Adequate arch support with shock-absorbing properties is ideal.

Individuals who suffer from hip osteoarthritis may benefit from a wide-fitting shoe with excellent shock-absorbing characteristics. Osteoarthritis often results in deformed foot joints, such that the foot becomes irregular with pressure points like bunions and hammertoes. Good arch support is also necessary. The correct shoe will reduce hip pain and significantly increase its function. A rocker bottom shoe can be of great benefit, as it helps one take off easily from the ground when walking.

Emerging research shows that there is a correlation between footwear and arthritis of the hip, knee and feet. A good shoe can change muscle activation and gait. Most sufferers complain of pain in certain points of the foot. These points include the heel, the arch and the ball. Orthotics can be used to remove weight-bearing pressure from these areas, thus improving step and stride and further reducing the amount of energy used while walking.

A rigid or soft orthotic can be used. Rigid ones are important in individuals with flat feet. They reduce foot loading and prevent deformities that may occur, like valgus positioning of the toes. Soft orthotics provide comfort; however, orthopedic and orthotic shoes do have some extra weight. Running shoes are a good substitute; they are lightweight and comfortable.

For patients with osteoarthritis of the hip, the disease also affects other joints, most commonly the knee. Lateral wedge and subtalar-strapped orthotics can be used in such cases. These have been shown to significantly reduce the muscle pull on the medial knee compartment, which is the most affected by osteoarthritis of the knee.

The fact that footwear can alleviate pain associated with arthritis suggests that footwear can also cause arthritis. In some studies, wearing high heels did not increase the risk of developing osteoarthritis, but they increased the risk of developing foot pain and lower back pain. The use of high heels, sandals and slippers in the present or past is correlated with greater chances of developing foot pain, women being more affected than men. Nonetheless, a good shoe can do so much for pain relief of hip arthritis.

Shoes of a low height (two inches and below) are recommended. Some shoes to check out are Hotter shoes, Cosyfeet, the Mark and Spencer foot glove, Simple Way shoes and Ecco shoes. See cosyfeet.com, hottershoes.com and widerfitshoes.co.uk.

Chapter 7: Hip arthroplasty

Total Hip Replacement

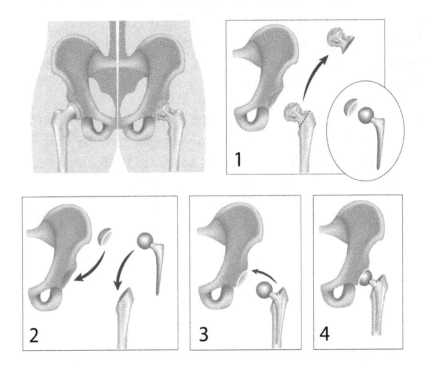

Arthritis of the hip is one of the common debilitating conditions that results in progressive disability. Disability in hip arthritis is associated with the inability to stand, walk, and perform activities such as running. As we have learnt, arthritis of the hip is progressive wearing off of the articular cartilage of the hip joint. These erosions of the joint surface result in bone-to-bone rubbing, which creates pain and reduced range of movement.

After arthritis of the hip has been diagnosed, the disease severity is graded. Very severe joints require surgery as an initial treatment at the time of diagnosis; however, most sufferers receive conservative therapy before surgery is planned.

Hip surgery can be open or arthroscopic. The choice of the kind of surgery to be performed depends on the type of surgery required. For instance, cleaning of the hip joint with removal of growing pannus on the articular surface can be done arthroscopically; however, a total hip replacement requires opening. Total hip replacement is a rapidly-growing procedure. It involves removing part of the femur head and the acetabulum, then replacing them with metal or plastic prostheses. Artificial joint prostheses can be made from all kinds of metals, metal alloys, plastic or ceramic. The material has to be non-allergenic, safe, and durable. After the procedure, aggressive physiotherapy is the key to effective hip replacement surgery. Post-surgery care is also crucial, since blood clots and infections can be dangerous complications.

1) What is hip arthroplasty?

Hip arthroplasty is a breakthrough procedure in the treatment of hip arthritis. It relieves pain, restores function and improves the quality of life. A British orthopedic surgeon, Sir John Charnley, is considered to be the father of total hip arthroplasty (THA). He designed the hip prosthesis and developed the fundamentals of the procedure. The US performs an estimated 300,000 THAs yearly.

For an individual to opt for THA as a treatment option, they ought to understand the risks of the procedure and the expected outcomes. A good candidate for THA would be a patient who will benefit from the procedure through reduced pain and improved hip function.

a) Risks of THA

- Infection

Infections are classified by the time at which they occur after surgery. Early onset is an infection that occurs within 3 months post-surgery. Delayed onset occurs between 3-12 months following a hip replacement. Late onset infections start at 12 months or more after a THA. Early onset infections could occur during the surgery itself, when infectious agents from the skin are introduced into the surgical wound with the implants. Staphylococcus aureus is the most common pathogen inoculated from such infections. Delayed and late infections may result when pathogens from another site of the body are transferred to the prosthesis via the blood, which is known as hematogenous spread. Whichever way the infection arises, they are a leading cause of THA failure.

Symptoms of an infection include: high temperature of 38 degrees Celsius or more, shaking, chills, a swollen, red joint, discharge from the surgical wound, and persistent hip pain.

Treatment of infections after THA requires multiple surgeries of debridement, implant removal, antibiotic beads insertion and removal, and prolonged antibiotic therapy. When the infection clears, another replacement surgery will be necessary. Unfortunately, chances of infection increase after a previous infection.

- Hip dislocation

A hip dislocation of the prosthesis can occur in 1 patient of every 20. These dislocations may happen due to improper joint angle calculations during surgery, squatting, and force at the knee which pushes the femur backwards. A hip dislocation requires immediate surgery to return it to its proper place.

- Loosening of the joint

This complication can occur at any time, but often happens 10 years or more after surgery. The bone around the implant on the femur becomes thin, allowing the implant to move within the bone. A patient will complain of instability of the joint during use. Revision of the implant by surgery is the best treatment, though not every patient is fit for a revision.

- Nerve and blood vessels injury

With surgery comes some risk of injury to other body tissues that are otherwise normal before surgery. The sciatic nerve, being located posterior to the hip, can have trauma intra-operatively. This will result in a foot drop and inability to use the lower limb post-surgery. Iatrogenic nerve and vascular injury often occurs with the use of tourniquets, as well as injuring a neurovascular bundle that has unusual anatomy.

- Wear and tear

Wear and tear of an artificial joint is common. When a young and active individual has a THA, with time, it is usually bound to wear out. Wear of the prosthesis happens when certain metals rub against each other. Therefore, it is a good preventative measure to make joints that have combinations of materials, like a metal and a plastic. Men often have more of the THA failures than women. Also, the younger the patient, the greater the chance of failure. Improper operating techniques also contribute to the rate of hip replacement failure. Non-cemented prostheses tend to fail more than cemented ones. Revision and replacement of the joint is necessary to restore function and relieve pain.

- Joint stiffness

Inadequate physio post-surgery may cause the development of fibrous tissues around the implant. These tissues restrict the joint range of motion and the joint function. Joint stiffness can be prevented by an aggressive exercise routine after a THA, medications and radiotherapy.

- Blood clots

Thrombus formation after surgery of long bones and hip replacements is a serious complication. Thrombus can be logged in the blood vessels of the lower limbs, known as deep vein thrombosis (DVT), or as a thrombus that is taken up to the lungs, or a pulmonary embolism (PE).

DVT signs include a swollen, tender, warm, red and painful lower limb. PE symptoms are breathlessness, gasping for air, a sharp chest pain and cough. Both these conditions are medical emergencies that require immediate treatment, otherwise death can occur.

To prevent this complication, anti-clot medications like heparin and Waafarin are usually given after THA. Individuals with a greater risk of developing thrombo-embolism, like obese individuals and the elderly, need close monitoring.

-Others

Other complications that can occur with THA include leg length discrepancies, fracture of the femur or hip bone, wound irritation with excessive scar formation and keloids, and failure to relieve pain.

b) Signs that THA might be necessary:

- Pain

-Functional limitation

- Joint stiffness

-Aged between 60-80 years

- Severe radiographic changes of the hip joint.

c) Factors that may make THA a less desirable option:

- Psychiatric patient

- Dementia

- Systemic infection

- Morbid obesity

- Vascular insufficiency

- Poor soft tissue coverage

- Ulcers

- Neuropathic hip disease, e.g. Charcot hip

2) How the procedure is done

a) Pre-op preparation
Before surgery, thorough preparations are carried out, including:

- Blood tests e.g. FBP

- A physician orders a general medical examination

- Medications like aspirin, anti-inflammatory drugs, herbal medicines and blood thinners are stopped 10 days prior to surgery

- The patient is advised to stop smoking 10 days before surgery.

- The anesthetist also performs an examination.

- The patient is counseled by a nurse, and answers a set of medical questions.

- The patient is given hospital clothes and takes a bath before surgery.

- The operation site is cleaned and shaved.

- The patient must abstain from any food or drink on the day of surgery.

b) Steps of the procedure
- The surgeon makes an incision over the hip to expose the joint.

- The acetabulum is prepared for prosthesis by a process called reaming. A reamer can be electric or manual. The reamer has a shape like the femur head, but has holes that can cut through cartilage and bone during the reaming process. The cartilage of the acetabulum is removed and the surface smoothed out. An artificial acetabulum component is then inserted. At times, this component is held in place by screws.

- The femur is then prepared. The arthritic head is cut and the bone prepared in such a way that it can allow the stalk of the femoral component to be inserted. After insertion, the stalk of the femoral component can be cemented in place by bone cement, or it can be tightly fit in, relying on new bone to form and fill in the small spaces, thus tightly securing the component to the femur.

- The femur head is then connected to the stalk. The femur head is often made from metal or ceramic.

- The femur head is then logged or reduced into the prosthetic acetabulum.

- Muscles and tissues are then closed, marking the end of the operation.

c) Post-op care
- After surgery, blood pressure, temperature, oxygen saturation and urine output are closely monitored.

- Post-op antibiotics are prescribed for 24 hours, 48 hours or, at times, 72 hours.

- Analgesics are also prescribed, but after 48 hours the pain is often minimal.

- Post-op x-rays are done to reveal the position of the hip after surgery. This x-ray is necessary to judge the success and position of the hip components, and also for future comparisons and references.

- Drains are removed from the wound after 24 hours. However, if the wound still has a lot of blood or fluid coming out, the drain can be left for another 24 hours. Wound dressing is done on a daily basis. By the second day after surgery, most patients are stable enough to be taken to the ward from the recovery room.

- A physiotherapist assists the patient to ambulate as soon as possible. They then plan an exercise routine for the patient, and teach them how to perform the exercises on their own.

- After 5-6 days post-surgery, a patient is discharged home and is to continue with physiotherapy at home.

- It is advised to use crutches for the first 2 weeks following surgery, then to walk with other aids for another 4-6 weeks.

- Stitches are removed 10-14 days after surgery.

3) Rehabilitation

Rehabilitation allows proper healing of the hip after THA. This includes lifestyle changes that are necessary to aid uninterrupted healing. Sleep with a pillow between your legs, as it increases comfort. This should be done during the first 6 weeks. During that same period, avoid bending your hip to 90 degrees, or bending while your foot is rotated inwards or outwards. Wear slip-ons inside the house to avoid bending to put on shoes. Grabbers and tongs can be bought to pick things up off the ground.

Wound care is of utmost importance. Daily wound dressing, with application of antimicrobial moisturizing cream, is suggested. High chairs are recommended in the dining room, and raising the toilet seat may also be helpful. Safety bars and handrails in the shower are handy. One is allowed to bathe once the wound has healed. If the house has a staircase, supporting rails can also be put in place. Loose rugs and electric cords should be removed from walking space. These may result in further injury if you are to fall.

Other lifestyle changes involve having a relative or family member over during the first weeks after surgery. It is during this period that you will require the most help with household chores. Attempt to eat all meals and follow a healthy, balanced diet. After any surgery, loss of appetite is common, but try by all means to eat well. After 3-6 weeks, one should be able to do normal, light activities. Through all this, daily exercise is a must. It is necessary to restore movement and to strengthen the hip.

Tips

❖ Avoid crossing legs over into a figure 4 or at the ankle.

❖ Do not bend your hip to a 90 degree angle.

❖ Do not turn your foot excessively, inwards or outwards.

❖ Take precautions to avoid falls and injury.

❖ Your dentist should be informed about your THA.

❖ Check with the surgeon for follow-up examination and advice.

4) How to use an artificial hip joint

One has to adapt to having an artificial hip, but it is something that you can be taught. Patients with total hip prosthesis may have the metal detector beep at airports. Carry an official document to show that you have had a hip replacement. A patient with hip implants may not use machines that have high magnetic power like MRI machines. Notify other doctors that you have had joint replacement surgery. A clicking sound may be heard as the joint is moved; this is something that one has to get used to, although it can be very annoying.

Maintain a healthy lifestyle. Gaining significant weight after total hip arthroplasty may compromise the implants. Some daily activities like driving cannot be performed soon after surgery; patients are advised to wait 3 months. Avoid carrying heavy things and performing high-intensity activities. Sexual activity can be resumed after 6 weeks, although you and your partner should take care to choose appropriate and comfortable positions. Remember to avoid bending the hip to 90 degrees or more.

Chapter 8: Other remedies for hip arthritis

1) Dietary treatment

Hip osteoarthritis is classified as ICD 10- M16 by the Center for Disease Control and Prevention. This condition, as well as other arthritis conditions including rheumatoid arthritis, reactive arthritis, post-traumatic arthritis, and gout arthritis, causes chronic hip pain but can benefit from dietary treatment. Treating hip arthritis with diet involves supplementing important elements through food.

The body requires a balanced diet with adequate nutritional value in order to repair injured tissues. Bones and cartilage contain calcium, phosphorus, magnesium, chondroitin and glucosamine. Vitamin D in its active form, known as calcitriol and calcidiol, work with the parathyroid hormone to control necessary metabolism within the skeletal system. A good hip diet for relieving hip arthritis should contain all of these minerals and vitamins. Some foods rich in these nutrients include broccoli, lentils, spinach, milk, egg whites, and mushrooms and should be included often in meals.

A vegan diet is preferred; however, it's not a necessity. The benefits of a vegan diet include weight loss and body mass maintenance. Vegan diets also reduce the inflammation associated with consuming meat, especially red meat. Animal fats contain vast amounts of polyunsaturated fatty acids, which support the development of diseases like arteriosclerosis and obesity. Avoiding meat altogether is ideal, however white meat like skinned chicken or fish are good alternatives to red meat.

Hip arthritis diets can also be made specific to the kind of arthritis that an individual sufferers from. Gout arthritis, for instance, involves the accumulation of uric acid crystals within the joints. Therefore, foods that lead to increased uric acid production such as meat should be avoided in the diet.

Some research studies suggest that hip arthritis sufferers should not eliminate any foods from the diet. However, I believe that an informed person who understands the pathogenesis of hip arthritis cannot help but be choosy.

A good diet for hip arthritis is one that enhances immunity and reduces inflammation. Fruits and vegetables will provide adequate vitamins; however, the fruit selection should not be of the high sugar kind such as grapes, bananas, and watermelon. If these fruits are to be included, their portions should be limited.

Vegetable based oils, like olive oil and sunflower oil, should be used in place of animal oils, with the exception of cod liver oil, which is beneficial. Vegetable oil based butters and margarines should also substitute the animal based varieties. In addition, a diet high in Omega 3 is known to reduce inflammation. Foods that are naturally high in Omega 3 are walnuts, soya beans, and flax seeds. Omega 3 can also be found in synthetic supplements of butter, oils, and tablets. Omega 3 has many benefits, including mood stimulation, memory improvement, and strengthening of hair and nails. Both Omega 3 and Omega 6 are usually synthetically added to foods, but for hip arthritis, one should include Omega 6 sparingly in the diet. Omega 6 is known to cause obesity and support inflammatory processes, both effects that one should avoid for effective hip arthritis treatment.

Certain herbs, drinks and teas also have a positive use in the treatment of hip arthritis. Cherry juice, green tea, chamomile tea, and white tea are great options for arthritis sufferers. Herbs such as cinnamon powder, the devil's claw root, ginseng, boswellia, capsicum, apple cider vinegar, and licorice are healthy additions to an arthritic diet. One should research different kinds of recipes that include these substances. Finding fun recipes that you like will make it easy for you to consume the foods for treating arthritis in the right quantities. Some substances can be applied directly onto the hip region after a bath, such as eucalyptus oil or a mustard powder paste. Keeping the joints warm by wearing warm, cotton based clothing is also helpful.

2) Yoga

Yoga is a method of holistic medicine. Regular practice improves the body's well being by integrating mind and body. For hip arthritis, yoga is a good alternative to traditional exercise, which may be too strenuous for arthritis sufferers. Yoga for beginners involves simple stretching activities that enhance strength, flexibility, and balance. Another holistic treatment that may be considered is t'ai chi.

Yoga originated in ancient India. The word yoga is Sanskrit, meaning "to unite". Yoga involves spiritual well-being, which provides benefits of improved mental well-being, emotional stability, and physical strength. Most people think that yoga is aimed only at improving flexibility, and that only individuals who are flexible can participate in yoga classes. This is not the case. Yoga is a broad practice encompassing strength, body posture, and body alignment. Yoga is safe, and through research, has been proven to be an effective form of exercising.

As with any physical exercise, yoga increases energy, happiness, and alertness. Due to this effect, individuals that suffer from chronic conditions like arthritis can benefit significantly from yoga. Exercise such as yoga reduces feelings of stress, anxiety and depression, resulting in overall mood enhancement. To date, there are only a few research studies that have been conducted on yoga's effects as a treatment for chronic arthritis, but the few that have been done have shown positive results.

Be sure to consult your GP before starting yoga sessions. Improper performance of yoga positions can lead to injury and body position anomalies over time. Therefore, great care should be taken during classes. Make sure that you learn to do the positions the correct way, from a qualified instructor. Yoga instructors, like physical therapists and doctors, require certification. Before you start any sessions, be sure your instructor is qualified and certified to teach yoga.

In a beginner's class, learn proper alignment for poses, how to relax, and develop the correct breathing techniques. According to the Arthritis Foundation, a study conducted by the John Hopkins University on 30 sedentary adults involved enrolling the subjects in 8 weeks of yoga classes. During and after the study, the subjects reported reductions in joint swelling and tenderness.

One of yoga's advantages is that if one knows how to perform it, it can be done anywhere—at the workplace, at the airport, or while waiting for a bus or train. Yoga can be fun if a friend or relative joins in on your sessions. It gives you both something to talk about, and the support will make sessions more enjoyable. When practicing yoga, always be aware of your body's current state. Listen to your body and recognize your limitations. Yoga is more of a focus exercise than a competitive one, so be gentle with every pose. Positions can be modified for individuals with significant limitations, such as those with severe arthritis. Your instructor can help you modify the poses to suit your needs. Here are some yoga positions to check out:

A) Cobbler's pose

1) Sit on the floor in an upright position, with your legs together and straight in front of you.

2) Bring the soles of your feet together, opening your knees to the sides.

3) Place your hands on your feet to fasten them in place, making sure that your elbows are pushed into your thighs.

4) Bend from the hips and lean forward, keeping your chest and chin straight.

5) Hold the position for 30 seconds, release, and return to the starting position.

B) Standing forward bend

1) Stand with your body straight, knees slightly bent, keeping your feet slightly apart.

2) Slowly bend forward from the waist, as far as is comfortable. Let your arms hang loosely towards the floor.

3) Hold the position for 6 seconds, then slowly come back up to the starting position.

4) Repeat the routine 5 or 6 times.

C) Diaphragmatic breathing

1) Stand in an upright position and place your hands over your abdomen.

2) Slowly take a deep breath, and watch your hands rise as you inhale.

3) Slowly exhale.

4) Do not force the breathing, take short breaths if needed.

5) Repeat 5 times.

Tip

Inhaling and exhaling quickly more than 15 times in a row can result in fainting due to hyperventilation. This routine is to be done slowly.

D) Chair

1) Stand in a straight position, legs together and arms by your sides.

2) Raise both arms overhead as you take a deep breath.

3) Slowly bring your arms down to your sides, squatting as if you are about to sit on a chair.

4) Hold the position for 5 seconds and then return to the starting position.

5) Repeat the routine 5 times.

Tip

Breathe gently and slowly through this routine.

E) Corpse roll

1) Lie straight on your back, with your legs wide apart.

2) Slowly roll your feet inwards, then outwards.

3) Repeat 10 times on each side.

Tip

This routine improves hip mobility by loosening the joints' internal and external rotation.

F) Downward Facing Dog

1) Kneel down on your hands and knees, keeping your back straight.

2) Straighten your legs to move your body upwards, making your body into an upside down V shape.

3) Move your feet a few steps back for a good stretch.

4) Suck your stomach in, and breathe deeply.

5) Hold the position for 4 minutes, and then return to starting position.

6) Rest for 3 seconds, and repeat the pose.

Tip

Chronic hip pain can also cause back pain. This exercise relaxes the back and shoulders.

G) Crescent Lunge

1) Stand with one leg in front of you, bent at a 90 degree angle.

2) Keep the other leg straight behind you.

3) Put your palms together, and raise your arms straight up.

4) Lean your head back, keeping your back straight and hips facing forward.

5) Hold the position for 5 seconds, release and return to a straight back.

6) Rest for 3 seconds and repeat the position 3 times.

Tip

This exercise stretches your hips, knees, and lower back.

H) Half Bow Pose

1) Lie on the floor on your stomach, keeping arms and legs straight.

2) Raise both your legs and arms off the ground, grabbing the right ankle with the right hand.

3) Keep the left arm and leg straight and off the ground.

4) Pull your ankle gently toward your buttock.

5) Hold the position for 5 seconds, and then release.

6) Repeat the pose with your left leg.

Tip

This exercise opens the chest and improves breathing

I) Boat Pose (for men)

1) Sit on the floor with your legs straight in front of you, keeping your back straight.

2) Lift both your legs off the ground, leaning backwards for balance.

3) Place both your arms straight in front of you, and hold the position for 3 seconds.

4) Bring your legs down to the ground and rest for a moment, then repeat the pose.

Tip

This exercise enhances thyroid, prostate, and gland function.

J) Hero Pose

1) Kneel down on your knees, keeping your body upright and arms straight by your sides.

2) Sit on your bent legs.

3) Lean forward, allowing your body to rest on your folded knees.

4) Keep your head at least 2 inches off the ground.

5) Hold the position for 5 seconds.

6) Return to an upright, seated position and rest for a few seconds.

7) Repeat the pose again.

Tip

This position stretches the knee joint. Hip arthritis often affects the knee joint.

K) Reclining Big Foot

1) Lay on your back, keeping your legs together.

2) Raise your right leg, keeping it straight.

3) Grab the raised right leg with the left hand, pulling to keep it straight.

4) Keep the right arm stretched straight and sideways.

5) Hold the position for 3 seconds.

6) Release the leg and return to the starting position.

7) Close your eyes and breathe deeply. Then repeat the pose, stretching the other side.

L) The Gate Pose

1) Kneel on the floor, with your right leg straight in front of you.

2) Keeping your body straight, bend sideways to the right, with your left arm raised straight in the air.

3) Hold the position and breathe deeply.

4) Breathe deeply as you return slowly to the starting position.

5) Switch the leg and arm, and repeat the pose.

M) Eagle Pose

1) Stand on one leg.

2) Wrap the other leg around the balancing leg.

3) Twist your arms around each other, so that the palms are back to back, and the thumb is directly under the small finger of the other hand, keeping your elbows at right angles.

4) Hold the position for 10 seconds, release, and stand up on both feet.

5) Rest for a few seconds, then repeat using the other leg and reversed hand position.

N) Tree Pose

1) Stand on one leg, with the other foot flat against the inner thigh of the standing leg (making the figure 4).

2) Stretch your arms straight up, and tilt your head backwards.

3) Hold the position for 5 seconds.

4) Return to starting position, then switch legs and repeat.

O) Camel Pose

1) Kneel on the floor, keeping your back straight.

2) Position your arms straight behind you and touch the bottom of your feet.

3) Drop your head backwards while arching your torso forward.

4) Breathe and hold the position for 5 seconds.

5) Return to the starting position.

118

6) Rest for a few seconds and repeat the pose 2 times.

P) Cobra Pose

1) Lie on your abdomen, keeping your legs together.

2) Using your straight arms along your sides for support, raise your chest off the ground.

3) Stretch as far as you can, and then hold the position for a few seconds.

4) Release the pose and lie back down.

5) Rest and repeat the pose 5 times.

Q) Reverse Cobbler Pose

1) Sit with your feet facing each other, keeping your knees out to the sides and flat on the floor.

2) Keep your torso straight.

3) Place your arms straight behind you to place your palms on the floor.

4) Hold the position for a few seconds.

5) Release and repeat the pose 3 more times.

R) Forward Bend

1) Sit with your legs together, keeping your body straight.

2) Lean forward and rest your chest on the outstretched legs.

3) Stretch your arms forward to touch your toes and rest your head on your knees.

4) Hold the pose for 5 seconds.

5) Release and repeat 5 times.

S) Locust Pose

1) Lie flat on your abdomen, keeping your legs and arms straight and parallel to the floor.

2) Raise both legs and torso off the ground, including your arms.

3) Hold the position for 10 seconds. Only your pelvis should be touching the floor.

4) Release and repeat the pose 4 times.

T) Double Pigeon Pose

1) Sit with your legs bent at the knee at a 90 degree angle, such that when you look between your legs you see a triangle shape.

2) Stretch your arms straight in front of you, placing your palms flat on the floor.

3) Lower your torso to rest your head on the floor.

4) Hold the position for 5 seconds, and then release.

5) Repeat the pose 3 times.

U) Three Faced Pose

1) Sit on the floor with one leg straight in front of you, and the other bent under your buttock.

2) Lean forward, resting your torso on your outstretched leg.

3) Grab your feet, and rest your chin on your knee.

4) Hold the position for 60 seconds and release.

Tip

This exercise stretches the knee and ankle joints. It also relieves leg swelling.

V) Happy Baby Pose

1) Lie flat on your back.

2) Bring your knees toward your stomach.

3) Grab your feet with both hands.

4) Separate your legs by pulling them to the side, positioning them just under your armpits.

5) Hold the position for 60 seconds.

W) Monkey Pose

1) Sit on the floor with legs as close to a 180 degree angle as you can.

2) Raise your arms straight up above your head, as far as you can reach.

3) Hold the position for 30 seconds.

Tip

This pose strengthens thighs and hamstring muscles, widening the hip and groin.

X) Garland Pose

1) Squat with your feet close together.

2) Keep your hands in a prayer position.

3) Move your legs apart, leaning your torso forward between your thighs.

4) Hold the position for 60 seconds.

5) Release the pose, return to standing, and rest.

Y) Fish Pose

1) Lie on your back, with your legs and arms straight.

2) Press your elbows firmly on the floor to lift your chest off the ground, relaxing your head backwards.

3) Hold the position for 60 seconds and release to starting position.

4) Repeat the pose 3 times.

Z) Lion Pose

1) Kneel on the floor, crossing your legs over each other at the ankles.

2) Sit back on your crossed legs.

3) Stretch your arms in front, palm down, with your fingers spread out.

4) Open your mouth wide, stretching your tongue out towards your chin.

5) Open your eyes wide open.

6) Breathe in through your nose, but breathe out loudly through your mouth, making a roaring sound.

7) Switch the position of your crossed legs and repeat the pose.

General yoga Tips

- ❖ Remove shoes before beginning. Yoga is performed barefoot.

- ❖ Beginners should arrive to the class early. Introduce yourself to the instructor and explain your condition.

- ❖ Be gentle with every pose.

- ❖ Stop if you feel any pain.

- ❖ Avoid hyper-extending the neck, back, and any other joints.

- ❖ Do not hold your breath during routines. Even if the routine is challenging, remember to breathe calmly!

- ❖ Wear comfortable clothes that are not too tight or too loose. One can buy specific yoga clothes, although this is not necessary.

- ❖ Have a stable mat for cushioning and to prevent slipping.

- ❖ Namaste—Namaste is a greeting done in yoga. The instructor bows his or her head whilst they place the hands on the chest and say "Namaste". Repeat as the instructor has done. Namaste is a Sanskrit word that means, "I honor you."

- ❖ Avoid leaving the class in the middle of sessions where everyone is trying to relax and find inner peace. Leave earlier before such routines if you really must leave.

❖ Bring a water bottle with you—hydrate frequently and adequately.

❖ If you are a beginner, practice yoga in a class at a fitness or yoga center. Home yoga is not recommended for beginners. But once you get acquainted to the practice, you can have home sessions by yourself.

3) The Alexander Technique

In life, we are often unaware of the behaviors and habits that cause us stress and hinder our ability to respond to stimuli normally. The Alexander Technique, devised nearly 100 years ago, is a method of education used to change bad habits.

Fredrick Mathias Alexander, a Shakespearean actor who would often lose his voice due to the habitual bending of the neck and head, created this technique. While performing, he would lose his voice or it would become raspy. Doctors did not know what was wrong with him. With careful self-observation, over time he discovered that tension during speech was causing his voice problem. When he worked to improve this habit, he noticed that his overall coordination also improved. The recurrent voice problem disappeared, and he established proper concepts and principles for his technique.

Individuals who suffer from chronic hip pain can benefit from using the Alexander Technique. The technique teaches individuals the best way to coordinate their musculoskeletal system. Other people such as athletes and dancers use the Alexander technique to enhance performance. Musicians also use it to train their vocal cords and breathing. Furthermore, this technique can help individuals become more alert and develop better control of their actions. Some might say that the Alexander technique balances one's psychology.

The basic concepts of this technique involve recognizing the undesirable habit first. An Alexander teacher will diagnose a bad habit. One can then appreciate why a certain habit is undesirable, and the feelings and sensations associated with the problem. Next, the individual learns how to inhibit these sensations, followed by instruction on how to correctly perform the action.

Similarly to Yoga, the Alexander Technique requires a private teacher. Alexander teachers study for about 3 years; they too need certification. Sessions are given on an individual basis and last for 30-60 minutes. No special attire is necessary; one can practice the technique in everyday clothing. The number of classes needed depends on the goals of the attendee. Most people take classes for 3-6 months, but some may take classes for more than a year. The Alexander Technique is a great way for people to learn about themselves. For more information, see www.amsatonline.org.

Summary

Hip arthritis is a growing concern worldwide that calls for immediate measures to reduce its increasing prevalence. Awareness of the risk factors of arthritis should be discussed in educational programs. Once people understand that risks like obesity, heredity, smoking, age, gender, and poor diet plans can result in the development of hip arthritis, they can best protect themselves throughout their lives. Hip arthritis is a debilitating condition and when it is diagnosed people should also be well aware of the self-help options available to alleviate pain and maintain function.

Hip arthritis is just one of the diseases that can cause pain in the hip area. Many other conditions including bursitis, pregnancy, piriformis syndrome, and hip flexor injuries can cause pain in the hip area. A doctor can best make a proper diagnosis of hip arthritis after a thorough physical examination and various medical tests. Some tests that are commonly performed include ultrasounds, X-rays, MRIs, CT-scans, and diagnostic arthroscopy. Blood tests such as ESR, CRP, and FBP are also routine for a diagnostic exam.

Once a diagnosis has been made, an individualized treatment plan is formulated. NSAID medications are often prescribed, along with the use of intra-joint injections of corticosteroids and hyaluronic acid. Aids like crutches and walkers can be used when the joint is severely tender and painful. Physical therapy is needed throughout treatment plans of hip arthritis. When the hip is tender, exercise is limited to simple stretches in order to maintain joint mobility and range of movement; otherwise, physical therapy may be used to strengthen and improve the balance of a joint. Physical therapy also offers other pain relief modalities such as shockwave therapy, hot and cold therapy, and ultrasound treatment.

Alternative methods of treatment such as acupuncture, t'ai chi, and yoga have significant benefits. Surgery is another option if pain persists for long periods of time and cannot be improved by conventional treatment methods. Hip surgery involves partial and total hip arthroplasty, corrective osteotomies, and joint debridement. Surgery can be performed as a "key hole" surgery, known as an arthroscopy or open surgery. Arthroscopy is recognized for its cosmetic qualities. Once the hip joint has been replaced, the individual must learn to live with the new joint. Physical therapy plays a great role in the success of a THA and should be encouraged aggressively after surgery to maximize recovery. Like any surgery, THA has risks that can result in failure of the procedure. In most cases, an individual who has had a total hip replacement is able to continue a fully active life.

This book has been thorough, but further reading on the topic is encouraged. To all hip arthritis sufferers: knowledge is power. Read as many informative guides as you can. Joining medical blogs online is also helpful. Here, people who suffer from hip arthritis gather and share ideas about how to best cope with the disease.

Published by IMB Publishing 2014

CPSIA information can be obtained
at www.ICGtesting.com
Printed in the USA
BVHW080806110819
555603BV00021B/789/P

9 781909 151963